Preventing Intellectual Disability
Ethical and Clinical Issues

This is the first book that covers comprehensively the difficult ethical issues involved in prevention of intellectual disability (learning disability, mental retardation). These issues are discussed both practically and theoretically in the light of four case examples drawn from real life. The cases demonstrate various issues raised by the concept of preventing intellectual disability, including definition, epidemiology, screening and genetic counselling. Two major approach models (reproductive autonomy and public health) are scrutinised, and the practical issues of prevention are examined closely with respect to three syndromes (Down, Fragile X and Aspartylglucosaminuria). The question 'Why should intellectual disability be prevented?' is examined thoroughly at each stage.

As a paediatrician and a philosopher, Dr Louhiala presents the issues in a way that is both user-friendly and philosophically sound.

Dr Pekka Louhiala lectures in medical ethics in the Department of Public Health at the University of Helsinki. He is a trained paediatrician with an ongoing clinical practice, and is also a trained philosopher.

Preventing Intellectual Disability

Ethical and Clinical Issues

Pekka Louhiala

Department of Public Health
University of Helsinki, Finland

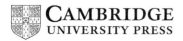
CAMBRIDGE
UNIVERSITY PRESS

PUBLISHED BY THE PRESS SYNDICATE OF THE UNIVERSITY OF CAMBRIDGE
The Pitt Building, Trumpington Street, Cambridge, United Kingdom

CAMBRIDGE UNIVERSITY PRESS
The Edinburgh Building, Cambridge CB2 2RU, UK
40 West 20th Street, New York, NY 10011–4211, USA
477 Williamstown Road, Port Melbourne, VIC 3207, Australia
Ruiz de Alarcón 13, 28014 Madrid, Spain
Dock House, The Waterfront, Cape Town 8001, South Africa

http://www.cambridge.org

First published 2004

Printed in the United Kingdom at the University Press, Cambridge

Typefaces Minion 10.5/14 pt., Formata and Formata BQ   *System* LaTeX 2$_\varepsilon$ [TB]

A catalogue record for this book is available from the British Library

Library of Congress Cataloguing in Publication data
Louhiala, Pekka.
Preventing intellectual disability : ethical and clinical issues / Pekka Louhiala.
        p.   cm.
Includes bibliographical references and index.
ISBN 0 521 82633 0 – ISBN 0 521 53371 6 (pb)
1. Mental retardation – Prevention – Moral and ethical aspects.   2. Mental retardation – Genetic aspects.
3. Learning disabilities – Prevention – Moral and ethical aspects.   4. Learning disabilities – Genetic aspects.
5. Genetic counseling – Moral and ethical aspects.   6. Genetic screening – Moral and ethical aspects.
7. Medical ethics.   I. Title.
RC570.L676 2003
616.85′8805–dc21   2003044032

ISBN 0 521 82633 0 hardback
ISBN 0 521 53371 6 paperback

Contents

Acknowledgements

This book is based on my Ph.D. thesis for the University of Wales Swansea. There is no doubt that, during the past eight years, the most important thing in my intellectual life has been my contact with the University's Centre for Philosophy and Health Care. Professor Zbigniew Szawarski, now in Warsaw, was my supervisor. He turned out to be a good *Doctor Vater* in many ways, always ready to give both intellectual and emotional support.

I am also very grateful to other members of the staff, who contributed to my work on various occasions. In particular, I want to mention Steven Edwards, who shared my interest in intellectual disability, and Martyn Evans, now in Durham, whose role in the development of my thinking about medical ethics and philosophy of medicine has been central. Both Steven and Martyn have also become my personal friends.

Many people have contributed to this work in its various phases. I particularly wish to thank Jarkko Hautamäki, Angus Clarke, Simo Vehmas, the GETHIC group (in particular Elina Hemminki, Piia Jallinoja and Arja Aro) and Linn Getz for their specific comments and Raimo Puustinen for his good company and general inspiration. Ms Georgianna Oja has very efficiently revised the language of the manuscript, for which I am grateful.

The late Professor Olli Heinonen, head of my department at the University of Helsinki at the time this research was launched, and his successor, Professor Mats Brommels, were always very supportive and encouraging.

I am grateful for the financial support provided by The Finnish Cultural Foundation, The Häme Foundation and The Helsingin Sanomat Foundation.

Last but not least, I wish to thank my dear family, my wife Liisa and my son V-P, for being there, not only for their emotional support but also for their clear-minded lay views on many of the issues covered in this book.

Introduction

Case 1

Sarah is a 35-year-old teacher. She has two daughters, 7 and 9 years of age, from her first marriage. Her second husband Tom is 42 years old and has no children of his own. Sarah is now pregnant at 17 weeks. The first visit to the maternity clinic took place at 11 weeks, and during that visit Sarah was told about serum screening for Down syndrome. The nurse described the syndrome and the screening procedure briefly and gave her a leaflet that presented the same issues in more detail.

At home Sarah and Tom studied the leaflet together and decided that she should have the screening test. Two weeks later the test was performed, and Sarah received the results during her next visit to the clinic.

The nurse explained to Sarah that her chances of having a baby with Down syndrome were 1 in 150. She also explained that, therefore, Sarah was considered to belong to a high-risk group and that a definitive diagnosis was possible though amniocentesis. However, the procedure itself would increase the risk of miscarriage by 1%.

At home Sarah explained the result to Tom and the dilemma they were now facing. If the risk estimate was valid, there was a 99.3% chance that the foetus did not have Down syndrome and a 0.7% chance that it did. If they wanted to be sure, the option was to undergo amniocentesis, but it would slightly increase the risk of miscarriage.

Sarah had asked for advice at her visit to the maternity clinic. In fact Sarah had asked the nurse what she would do in a similar situation. The nurse had been very sympathetic but refused to answer Sarah's question. She had explained, firstly, that she was in a different situation in her life and could not give a definitive answer to such a question. Secondly, it was against the ethical rules of her profession to answer such questions. However, she would fully support the couple, whatever they chose to do.

Case 2

Tina is a 28-year-old laboratory assistant who has just learned that she is pregnant. Both Tina and her partner Harry are happy about the news. It is Tina's first pregnancy and also the first child for Harry.

Tina has a younger brother Kevin, who is 22 years old and intellectually disabled. The disability is mild and its cause is fragile X syndrome. Kevin's diagnosis was confirmed when he was 6 years old. Currently Kevin is still living with his parents and he works in a sheltered workshop.

Because Tina is 6 years older than her brother, she has been very much involved in his care. Kevin has been rather healthy, but there were moderately serious behavioural problems in adolescence. The adult years have, however, been stable in this sense, and the relationships between the family members are warm.

Tina had been tested many years ago and found to be a carrier of the fragile X syndrome. She knows very well what this result means. The probability for intellectual disability in her offspring is considerable, high for boys and low but not insignificant for girls. In fact, the level of intellectual functioning tends to be lower in future generations with the fragile X genotype.

Tina and Harry discuss their situation with their primary care physician, who also knows Kevin very well. The doctor uses the term 'risk' when he describes the dilemma, but Tina, especially, is not very comfortable with the word. If she has a son, his intellectual capacity may resemble Kevin's. However, there is a chance that it may be considerably lower or higher. In the case of a girl the chances for significant intellectual disability are small.

Although Tina is worried about the situation, she tends to think that she would not have an abortion, whatever the result of the test on the foetus would be. Harry is much more distressed, and he finds the idea of continuing the pregnancy with a male foetus with fragile X syndrome almost impossible.

Case 3

Aspartylglucosaminuria (AGU) is a rare inborn metabolic disease leading slowly to severe intellectual disability in adulthood. It is inherited as a recessive trait, and the cases have been found almost exclusively in Finland. The prevalence of the AGU gene is approximately 1:30 in eastern and northern Finland and slightly lower in other parts of the country.

The disease itself is rare, two to four affected children being born each year in the whole of Finland. The gene responsible for AGU has been found, and there is a relatively inexpensive test for it.

Some physicians suggest that testing for the AGU gene should be introduced to routine maternity care in eastern and northern Finland because (1) although rare, the disease causes a significant burden for both the families and society, this burden being mainly psychological for the families and economic for society; (2) there is a reliable test for the responsible gene; and (3) the attitudes of the population are positive towards genetic testing for severe diseases.

How should the health authorities respond to the request?

Case 4

A newborn baby (later to be known as Baby Jane Doe) was noted to have Down syndrome and oesophageal atresia (i.e. a condition requiring prompt surgical intervention to enable feeding). An obstetrician noted the baby's condition and consulted a paediatrician. The latter again consulted another paediatrician. The doctors disagreed about appropriate care.

The obstetrician recommended that the baby stay at the hospital and be kept comfortable and free of pain. The paediatricians suggested transfer to another hospital, where surgical repair of the atresia would be possible. Mr Doe had sometimes worked closely with Down syndrome children and was of the opinion that such children never have a minimally acceptable quality of life. His wife shared the opinion, and therefore they decided to follow the suggestion of the obstetrician. Baby Jane Doe had comfort care and died of hunger one week later (Kuhse and Singer 1985).

These examples describe, from different points of view, situations in which the prevention of *intellectual disability*, actual or potential, is considered. The cases also reflect several ethical problems related to intellectual disability and its prevention. The degree of parental autonomy and the role of the medical community are crucial in all of the cases, although the emphasis in cases 1, 2 and 4 is more on the individual level and in case 3 it is on the societal level. The question of quality of life, both of the individuals in question and their families, is also relevant in all the cases. Case 1 deals with probabilities and risks and how people understand their meaning in particular cases.

I shall return to all of these cases and also introduce some new ones later. Let us, however, concentrate for a while on case 4, which received much attention and has also been widely discussed in medical, ethical and lay media.

The case of Baby Doe was not at all unique as such. Similar cases have taken place and will take place all over the world; in fact in many parts of the world a surgical alternative is not even possible. What was unique was the sequence of events that followed. A detailed description can be found, for example, in Kuhse and Singer (1985), and I shall only briefly summarise it.

When the management of the Bloomington Hospital heard of the case, they intervened and contacted the local court, where the parents were judged to have the right to choose 'a medically recommended course of treatment for their child in the present circumstances' (i.e. the passive way suggested by the obstetrician) (Kuhse and Singer 1985, p. 13). The local County Department of Public Welfare was appointed as the guardian of Baby Doe. The Department decided not to appeal, but the County Prosecutor's office took action when the infant was 4 days old.

Another judge refused to order intravenous feeding to keep Bay Doe alive, and the State Supreme Court was asked to intervene, and by a 3 to 1 vote the ruling of the lower court was overturned. Baby Doe's life ended on the day that emergency intervention was sought from the United States Supreme Court.

Among the first to react to the case was the right-to-life movement, but soon influential newspapers also deplored the decision 'to allow a helpless Down's syndrome infant to starve to death' (Kuhse and Singer 1985, p. 14.). President Reagan's administration also reacted very soon and proposed so-called 'Baby Doe regulations'. According to these regulations handicapped infants should have access to any medical and surgical treatment and nutritional sustenance available, and the handicap could not be a contraindication of such care. Several earlier versions of the regulations were struck down, but the final ones came into effect in October 1984.

The regulations affected practices, the changes in which became evident in a survey done among American neonatologists (Kopelman *et al.* 1988). Three out of four respondents believed that the regulations were not necessary to protect the rights of handicapped infants, and two out of three believed that the regulations interfered with parents' rights to determine the course of action that was in the best interest of their children. When the respondents were presented hypothetical cases of severely handicapped newborns, up to 32% stated that Baby Doe regulations required care (i.e. maximal life-prolonging treatment) that was not in the best interest of the child. One of the cases was trisomy 13 syndrome, which is a severe malformation syndrome leading to early death. Major textbooks in paediatrics recommend only comfort care for these infants.

The case of Baby Doe illustrates again the many dimensions and complex issues that can arise from a single case. The discussion has concentrated on the conflict between parental rights on one hand and the rights of the baby and society on the other. However, some factual details in the case have been disregarded. One such detail was the attitude of Mr and Mrs Doe towards Down syndrome children.

Mr Doe was a schoolteacher, and he had sometimes worked closely with Down syndrome children. He and his wife were of the opinion that such children *never had a minimally acceptable quality of life* (Kuhse and Singer 1985, p. 12, my italics). Since this opinion was apparently crucial when decisions concerning care were made, it is important to examine its validity.

American society in general, and the health care system in particular, differ from those in northern and western Europe. However, it is not probable that the life of Down syndrome children in the early 1980s essentially differed on the other side of the Atlantic. The quality of life of Down syndrome children is certainly affected by intestinal malformations in some, heart defects in some, and so forth. However, Mr Doe's belief that '[they] never had a minimally acceptable life' is false. Neither experience from daily life nor scientific evidence suggests that the quality of life of Down syndrome children would be so severely compromised.

It is highly questionable whether these kinds of prejudices should form a basis on which problems of life and death can be solved. We can imagine a situation in which a child would have diabetes and the parents would think that the quality of life of this child could never be acceptable. Here it is obvious to anyone that the parents are wrong.

What Mr and Mrs Doe were certainly also thinking of were the quality of life of the infant after surgical correction of the oesophageal atresia and the quality of life of the family as a whole. These considerations make their choice more understandable, but still the role of the doctors involved with the case is worth scrutinising. Two paediatricians suggested transfer to another hospital for surgery while three obstetricians recommended that Baby Doe stay in Bloomington. The obstetricians were, of course, aware of the consequences. One can ask which of the two groups of doctors knew more about Down syndrome and the life of families with such children. The answer is clear. Paediatricians meet such children constantly in their work, and obstetricians do not. In fact, they are often involved in screening programmes involving their prenatal diagnoses.

I have discussed the case of Baby Doe to illustrate some of the issues analysed more deeply in the following chapters. The case also illustrates the necessity for a very detailed description of the events of an actual case. In this particular case, the parents' view on the quality of life of people with Down syndrome turned out to be the crucial issue.

The starting point of this book is the multitude of difficult moral issues that arise in the context of the cases described in the beginning of this chapter. What follows will be related to these problems, sometimes very closely, sometimes more remotely.

Chapter 2 examines the concept of intellectual disability. Firstly, various terms used to describe the phenomenon are presented. Secondly, the important underlying concept of *intelligence* and its measurement are discussed. Thirdly, a very influential definition by the American Academy of Mental Retardation (AAMR) is presented. Fourthly, the relationships between intellectual disability and health are discussed in light of Christopher Boorse's and Lennart Nordenfelt's theories of health.

Chapter 3 summarises key issues in the *epidemiology* of intellectual disability. Various epidemiological research strategies yield different results, which, however, complement each other and can be used for different purposes. The causes and epidemiological trends of intellectual disability are also briefly described in this chapter.

In Chapter 4 the concept of *prevention* and its three levels are first defined. Then, the question '*Why should intellectual disability be prevented*' is briefly introduced. Thirdly, attitudes towards the intellectually disabled throughout history are described. Fourthly, the *labelling* of individuals as intellectually disabled and the consequences of this labelling are discussed. The chapter closes with a description of actual strategies for preventing intellectual disability.

The use of *prenatal diagnosis* and *screening* is often related to the prevention of intellectual disability. Chapter 5 discusses in detail the complex ethical issues of these practices. Firstly, the history, methods and indications of prenatal diagnosis are described. Secondly, the two major models for justifying the practices, the reproductive autonomy model and the public health model, are thoroughly scrutinised. Thirdly, the chapter deals with some other critical issues in prenatal diagnosis and screening. These are the slippery slope argument, the relationship between prenatal diagnosis and eugenics and the impact of the practices on the disabled in general.

The topic of Chapter 6 is *genetic counselling* (i.e. the activity between a health professional and an individual, or a couple or a family, in which diseases or conditions of genetic origin are discussed). Issues of genetic counselling are highly relevant to the main topic of this book, since the most complex ethical issues in the prevention of intellectual disability are related to conditions of genetic origin. The chapter deals firstly with the goals of genetic counselling and then with successful counselling situations. Thirdly, the advantages and disadvantages of directive and non-directive counselling are examined thoroughly. Fourthly, some characteristics of good genetic counselling are formulated. Finally, *geneticisation*, the tendency to describe more and more of the phenomena of life in terms of genes and DNA (deoxyribonucleic acid) is described and analysed.

Chapter 7 is the philosophical core of this book. It examines in detail the issue that was briefly introduced in Chapter 4: *why* should intellectual disability be prevented. The following main arguments are defined and scrutinised: (1) the eugenic argument; (2) the foetal-wastage argument; (3) the family burden argument; (4) the societal burden argument; and (5) the quality of life argument.

Another major philosophical issue, the *moral status* of intellectually disabled individuals, is dealt with in Chapter 8. Mary Ann Warren's multi-criterial account of moral status provides the framework of reference. Moral status before individual birth and after birth is analysed and the relevance of these analyses for intellectual disability is discussed.

After these two chapters with more philosophical content, Chapter 9 comes back to more practical issues and examines the ethics of prevention in practice. Down syndrome, fragile X syndrome and aspartylglucosaminuria, a rare recessive condition found mostly in the home country of the author, are used as examples.

In the conclusive chapter (Chapter 10), I return to the four cases presented in the very beginning of my book. The cases are examined in light of all the analyses presented in the preceding chapters.

Finally, a few words about the terminology used. In the beginning of the preparation of this book, I used the term 'mental retardation' to refer to the topic. It is a term very widely used, especially in the North American context. In the final stages of writing, however, I changed my mind and decided to use the term 'intellectual disability' instead. There are two reasons for this decision. Firstly, in very many cases no retardation actually takes place. Secondly, the problems these people usually have concern more their intellectual functioning, rather than their total mental functioning. Loving, for example, is a mental function, and most people with intellectual disability are as able to love as those of us with better intellectual capacity. In fact, they have also been characterised as 'congenitally unable to hate'.

On the definition of intellectual disability

Various terms referring to intellectual disability (ID) have been used, and they reflect both the times and the context of their use. In fact, it has been argued that the terms seem to have a 'half-life' of acceptability (Kopelman 1984). In their article on the definition and classification of mental retardation, Zigler *et al.* (1984, p. 215) stated that 'without a clear and universally accepted definition of mental retardation, efforts to understand its nature and to improve the lives of retarded persons must be seriously compromised'. (I use the term 'mental retardation' when I refer specifically to, for example, articles or the American classification using the term.) While it is true that there is no general agreement on the definition, it is, however, not clear whether a single and universal definition is a preferable goal. The amount to which any solution would help improve the lives of the intellectually disabled is also questionable.

For example, the terms 'moron', 'imbecile' and 'idiot' were originally introduced as technical terms to cover the levels of ID. Table 2.1 lists some of the terms that have been used during recent years.

The problems of the definition of ID have been dealt with at length in some medical and psychological texts. On the contrary, philosophical texts that deal with ID present poor definitions or no definition at all (Boddington *et al.* 1991). Philosophical work 'tends to gravitate toward considerations of either the very severe or the very mild forms of handicap, where difficulties of definition and questions of ethical justification are possible to present as less problematic' (Boddington *et al.* 1991, p. 78). Sometimes people with ID are mistakenly put into the same category as 'lunatics' or are referred to as 'human vegetables' (Boddington *et al.* 1991). It is also common that they are referred to as sick persons, especially among lay and medical people (Kurtz 1977).

Since terms related to ID must serve many purposes, it would perhaps be best to accept that a universal definition can never be attained. In the context of law, for example, the limits of control or benefit must be defined, in epidemiological research an exact quantitative definition is necessary, educators need their own

Table 2.1. Intellectual disability: current and past terminology

feebleminded	
moron	
imbecile, idiot	
mental retardation	mentally retarded
mental handicap	mentally handicapped
mental deficiency	mentally deficient
learning disabilities	learning disabled
intellectual impairment	intellectually impaired
intellectual disability	intellectually disabled
mental disability	mentally disabled
intellectually challenged	

terms, parents and client groups also have their own, and so on (Fryers 1992). The aim of this chapter is to discuss the conceptual problems related to the definition of ID, with special reference to the concepts of intelligence, normal and health.

Intelligence and intellectual disability

The definitions of ID are based on the concept of *intelligence* either exclusively or in a way that includes other criteria as well. The nature of intelligence is a controversial topic that has received wide attention throughout the history of philosophy and psychology.

A chapter on intelligence in the *Oxford Companion to Philosophy* (Honderich 1995, p. 411) opens with the following sentence: 'A family of intellectual traits, virtues and abilities occurring in varying degrees and concentrations'. Although it is not claimed to be a definition, this description demonstrates the problems inherent in many definitions of intelligence in that it assumes that we can precisely define and measure intellectual phenomena. But it is not so.

In the context of this chapter it is not possible, or necessary, to describe at length the controversies around the concept of intelligence. However, I shall give a brief overview on various theories as they are described in Robert J. Sternberg's *Metaphors of Mind – Conceptions of the Nature of Intelligence* (1990).

Metaphors of intelligence

Sternberg's main theme is that theories of intelligence are guided by underlying metaphors of the mind. If we are to understand theories and their interrelation, we have to understand the underlying metaphors. The question 'What is intelligence?'

turns into 'What is intelligence as viewed from the standpoint of a particular metaphor?' As with stipulative definitions, metaphors are not right or wrong, but they are more or less useful for various purposes (Sternberg 1990, p. 9).

Sternberg describes seven major metaphors of intelligence, four looking at the relation of intelligence to the internal world of the individual (the geographic, computational, biological and epistemological metaphors), two looking at the relation of intelligence to the external world of the individual (the anthropological and sociological metaphors) and one looking at the relation of intelligence to both the internal and the external worlds of the individual (the systems metaphor).

The *geographic* metaphor views a theory of intelligence as a map of the mind. The first representatives of this metaphor were the phrenologists, who related mental abilities to cranial bumps. Early in the twentieth century the metaphor of a map became more abstract and less literal, and new tools, like factor analysis, were invented for the study of intelligence. The inventor of this method, Charles Spearman, proposed two kinds of factors of intelligence: general and specific. For Spearman the general factor g, which he described as mental energy, was the basis of intelligence.

The geographic metaphor flourished in the first half of the twentieth century, and the theory of psychometric testing and measuring was developed in great detail. According to Sternberg, the main reasons for scepticism against it were (1) its limited ability to describe mental processes; (2) the difficulties involved in testing factor-analytic models against each other or to falsify them; and (3) the basing of the understanding of intelligence on individual differences (Sternberg 1990, pp. 109–10).

The development of computer science and computer technology gave rise to the *computational* metaphor, which analogises the processes of the mind to the software of a computer. Because the computational metaphor of intelligence was generated largely as a response to the geographic one, it focused on questions of process and on commonalities across people and processing. Individual differences received minor attention or none at all.

Sternberg criticised the computational theorists for not making the similarity between computer programs and human intelligence clear and not taking into account what people in various parts of the world mean by intelligence.

The *biological* metaphor seeks to understand intelligence in terms of the functioning of the brain. Assumptions about the correlation between neurophysiology and the mind are based on data from studies on brain-damaged individuals and on electrophysiological (like electroencephalography) and metabolic (like positron emission tomography) studies on healthy people. Research based on the biological metaphor has produced a vast amount of data in which various brain functions are related to cognition in general and to intelligence in particular.

The interpretation of the results of this research is not straightforward, however. Correlation does not imply causation, and, even if there is a causative link, the direction of the causation cannot be inferred on the basis of the relation only. The interpretation has often been that a biological phenomenon in the brain is the cause of a mental state, but this reductionistic view involves philosophical presuppositions. As a matter of fact, recent studies have shown, for example, that psychotherapy can produce changes in brain function that can be demonstrated with positron emission tomography (Fricker 1996).

The *epistemological* metaphor of intelligence draws heavily on the philosophy of knowledge. Its main representative was Jean Piaget, who created a well-known theory of the periods of development of the child, beginning with the sensorimotor period and ending with the formal-operational period. Piaget saw the function of intelligence as that of adaptation, which includes assimilating the environment into one's own structures (physiological or cognitive) (Sternberg 1990).

Piaget's ideas have had a profound influence on psychology, and generally his theory of the major stages of development has been accepted. His followers and critics have, however, shown severe defects in his theory. He has described carefully the development of formal and logical thought but not, for example, intuitive or aesthetic thought. Yet the latter are important parts of intelligence. It has also been shown that there may be different routes of development, and children may accomplish tasks at earlier ages than those suggested by Piaget. Piaget seems also to have largely ignored individual differences.

Representatives of the *anthropological* metaphor think that the concept of intelligence cannot be the same in different cultures, because what it takes to adapt in one culture is quite different from what it takes to adapt in another. The extreme wing, the radical cultural relativists, rejects any psychological universals across cultures.

The introduction of the anthropological metaphor has prevented theory and research from being totally Western-oriented. We may have a tendency to think that people in other cultures end up doing what is done in the West, if only not so well. Fieldwork has, however, shown that developmental patterns reflect the environment in which the child grows. For example, African infants show superior early sensorimotor development relative to Western infants.

As Sternberg noted, 'the anthropological metaphor provides a needed counterbalance' to the metaphors referring to the internal world of the individual (Sternberg 1990, p. 15). It has, however, the danger of going to the other extreme and neglecting the relevance of what is *inside* the individual.

Another metaphor, which concentrates on the relationship between intelligence and the external world of the individual, is the *sociological* metaphor. Where Piaget tended to view intelligence as moving from the inside outward, the Russian psychologist Lev Vygotsgy viewed it as moving from the outside inward. The sociological metaphor does not differ very much from the anthropological one; only the emphasis of research is different. Where the anthropologically oriented concern themselves with how culture affects intelligence, the sociologically oriented focus on the socialisation processes in which culture affects the development of intelligence.

The limitations of metaphors focusing on the internal *or* external world have led to the development of theories that try to include both aspects. Sternberg referred to these theories as using the *systems* metaphor. For example, Gardner proposed that intelligence is not a single thing, but, instead, there exist multiple forms of intelligence like linguistic, logico-mathematical, spatial, musical, bodily kinaesthetic, interpersonal and intrapersonal. These forms of intelligence are independent of each other, but they do interact. Sternberg himself has suggested a triarchic theory of intelligence, in which he distinguishes between three basic kinds of information-processing components, i.e. metacomponents, performance components and knowledge acquisition components. Metacomponents are higher-order processes used to 'plan what one is going to do, to monitor it while one is doing it, and to evaluate it after it is done' (Sternberg 1990, pp. 268–9). Performance components are lower-order processes that execute the instructions of the meta-components. Knowledge acquisition components are used to learn how to do what the metacomponents and performance components actually do. Thus Sternberg's theory actually consists of three interrelated subtheories. In the introduction to his book, Sternberg compresses as follows: ' . . . I define intelligence as consisting of those mental functions purposively employed for purposes of adaptation to, and shaping and selection of, real-world environments' (Sternberg 1990, p. 6).

Measuring intelligence

The measurement of intelligence has occurred mainly in the context of the geographic metaphor. As a matter of fact, intelligence testing and factor analysis – the basic methodology behind the metaphor – grew up together (Sternberg 1990).

In 1905 Binet and Simon published what is generally regarded as the first test of intelligence (Binet and Simon 1905, reprinted in Rosen *et al.* 1976). Its purpose was to identify children who were unlikely to benefit from the public education system of France. The intention of the testing process was to provide such children with a more suitable form of education (Berger and Yule 1985). At that time the terminology was in a state of confusion, for example, 'one imbecile in the first certificate, is marked idiot in the second, feeble-minded in the third, and degenerate in the fourth' (Binet and Simon 1905, p. 332).

Binet and Simon deliberately distanced themselves from two earlier scholars in the field, namely, Galton and Cattell, who had created a variety of psychophysiological tests, which they thought measured intelligence (Sternberg 1990). According to Binet and Simon, 'to judge well, to comprehend well, to reason well, these are the essential activities of intelligence' (Binet and Simon 1905, cited by Sternberg 1990, p. 74). To criticise the psychophysiological view on intelligence, Binet cited the example of Helen Keller, who could be expected to score high on, for example, tests of judgement but very low on psychophysiological tests.

The starting point of Binet and Simon was highly practical, but they were not atheoretical in their approach to intelligence. On the contrary, they developed a sophisticated theory – more so than many of their followers in the field of intelligence testing (Sternberg 1990).

Binet and Simon's test was a starting point for a long tradition of psychological testing for which the *intelligence quotient* (IQ) became a central concept. In the early tests IQ was defined as a *rate*, which included the factors mental age (MA) and chronological age (CA). The intellectual level of the individual was defined by MA, which was obtained with intelligence tests. IQ was then derived by dividing MA by CA and multiplying the result by 100.

IQ has remained a key concept in testing, but calculating it with the means of MA and CA proved to be problematic (Sternberg 1990). For example, the CA of a person does not affect his or her performance on tests, but it is probably highly related to social behaviour and interests. Zigler *et al.* (1984) gave the following example: we would hesitate to tell a 7-year-old with an average IQ to catch a bus and go downtown, but this task could well be within the ability of a 25-year-old intellectually disabled person with an MA of 7. Furthermore, mental age begins to slow in growth around 15 years of age, and causes serious problems for interpreting the test results after that age. For these and other reasons, the IQ in modern tests is computed on the basis of relative performance within a given age group (Sternberg 1990). The test scores have been standardised to have a mean of 100 and a standard deviation of 15 or 16. Such standardisation makes comparisons between scores and comparisons among the general population easy and meaningful. Thus current IQ scores are actually not quotients at all.

Later (I have not been able to trace the first occasion), it became typical to define ID in terms of the standard distribution of intelligence. At the turn of the twentieth century it was thought that IQ is distributed *normally* (i.e. according to the Gaussian curve) (Fig. 2.1).

Individuals whose IQ was below some point on this curve were defined as intellectually disabled. The most commonly used cut-off point for ID has been two standard deviations (SD) below the mean. The following definition has been widely used, for example, in epidemiological research:

Definition 1
A person is intellectually disabled if he or she falls below two standard deviations in a standardised intelligence test.

In most intelligence tests one SD is 15 points, and therefore an IQ of 70 has become the borderline defining ID.

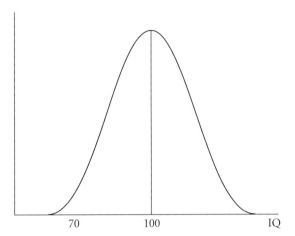

Figure 2.1   Standard distribution of intelligence.

Choosing two standard deviations is, of course, purely a matter of convention. In fact, it has been suggested that all individuals with IQs below *one* SD would comprise the group intellectually disabled, which would mean 16% of the population, not 2.3% as with the preceding definition.

The definition of ID based solely on IQ may serve its purpose when the aim is to obtain quantitative information concerning, for example, the number of individuals in need of special services. It is, however, far from adequate in describing individuals and their needs.

The constancy of IQ along the life cycle is another controversial matter. It has been suggested that the IQ of an individual can vary as much as 50 points (Hunt 1961). On the other hand, some researchers claim that for most people, IQ remains relatively stable.

It was noted as early as 1914 that the original assumption of the distribution of intelligence (as presented in Fig. 2.1) includes a fundamental error (Hagberg 1992). Large population tests have revealed that there are far more people at the lower end of the curve than could be expected from the Gaussian distribution. The prevalence of severe ID (IQ < 50) has, in several studies, been around 0.4%, although in the theoretical normal distribution it would be only 0.05% (Fryers 1984).

As an explanation for the excess of individuals with very low IQs, it has been suggested that there are actually two distributions of intelligence: one for the vast majority of people, for whom intelligence is a result of interaction between genes and the environment, and the other for the minority with organic damage (Figs 2.2a and 2.2b). (Figure 2.2a presents the peak at the lower end, as it has been presented in several texts (e.g. Zigler *et al.* 1984), but it is not at all clear that intelligence is normally distributed among those with suspected organic damage. Therefore the presentation in Fig. 2.2b may reflect the actual distribution better at the lower end.)

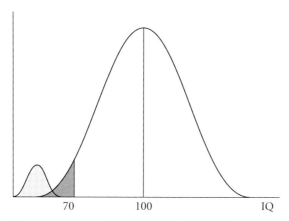

Figure 2.2a Two-group approach to intellectual disability, as presented, for example, by Zigler *et al.* (1984).

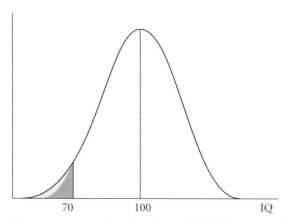

Figure 2.2b Two-group approach to intellectual disability: suggestion for the distribution at the lower end.

In any individual, genes play some role in determining intelligence, although there is no consensus in the scientific community as to what extent. In fact, a heated discussion still continues today after the publication of *The Bell Curve* (Herrnstein 1994), in which the author argues for a strong genetic basis for IQ. Nobody, however, denies that the environment has an important influence as well. As Zigler *et al.* (1984, p. 219) wrote: 'Whatever genes one inherits for intelligence (the genotype), the phenotype expression will be higher if the person experiences a good rather than a terrible environment.'

A recent review article in *Science* (Wickelgren 1999) describes research that swings the pendulum again towards the environment. Firstly, new results support the idea that racial differences in IQ are not genetically determined. Secondly, early speech input has been found to have a dramatic effect on the development of a child's language skills. Thirdly, a study comparing children born in the first nine months of one year to those born in the last three months of the same year showed a mean IQ difference of 3.5 points. This difference was entirely environmental since it was due to the fact that the former group entered school one year earlier.

Whatever the genetic basis for intelligence, it is not determined by a single gene but by several interacting genes, the number of which may be very large. For example, a five-gene model may explain the variation in IQ between 50 and 150 (between −3 SD and +3 SD) (Zigler *et al.* 1984). Although the model is artificial, it is in accordance with empirical findings concerning persons with very low IQs (below 50), who almost always show evidence of organic damage. Thus there must be another distribution for these persons, in whom the biological apparatus required for intelligence has been damaged pre-, peri- or postnatally.

For severe ID the proportion of people without organic damage is very low. On the other hand, the majority of the people with mild ID belong to the lower end of the normal curve (i.e. no damage can be shown for them). The latter group has been referred to as 'familially retarded' or 'retarded due to psychosocial disadvantage' (Zigler *et al.* 1984). By definition, there must be a group of people at the lower end; therefore these labels may be misleading. In this book, I refer to these people as *minus variants*, which is the term used also in the context of growth disorders.

For an individual it may be difficult or impossible to say whether he or she is a minus variant or has organic damage, which cannot be shown with current technology. As groups, however, the minus variants and those with brain damage show some differences. Members of the latter group often carry physical features or handicaps which differentiate them from others, while members of the former group do not. Those with organic damage often have siblings with a normal IQ, while minus variants have parents or siblings with IQs below average. This difference may influence the self-image of the children, as the child with organic ID feels different from other people in the family (Zigler *et al.* 1984). It has also been pointed out that a minus variant is most likely to be born to a family with low socio-economic status, while brain damage occurs more evenly across all levels of income (Zigler *et al.* 1984).

It may seem that the statistical definition of a phenomenon is value neutral. If we look, for example, at the distribution of height within a certain population, we obtain a curve, that at least roughly resembles the Gaussian curve. We then call the individuals 'short' whose height is below −2 SD on that curve. Is this a value-neutral judgement? No, because the very idea of having a group of short people contains a notion of 'shortness' as a deviant from 'normal'. In his book *On the Normal and the Pathological*, Georges Canguilhem described the nature of these concepts somewhat aphoristically: '. . . the pathological must be understood as one type of normal, as the abnormal is not what is not normal, but what constitutes another normal' (Canguilhem 1978, p. 119).

Table 2.2. The varieties of normal: words and expressions, which can replace 'normal' (modified from Gräsbeck 1995)

1. Ordinary, usual, everyday
2. Typical, characteristic
3. Mean, average
4. Gaussian, fitting the Gaussian distribution
5. Lies in the area x ± 2 SD
6. Does not statistically differ from healthy reference population
7. Physiological, reference, control
8. Optimal, ideal, good, not pathological
9. Not dangerous, harmless, trivial
10. Suitable, fits the norm(s), adequate
11. Recommended
12. Perpendicular

It should be noted here that the use of the word 'normal' is not at all unambiguous. If we specify that 'normal height' means exactly that one's height is between −2 SD and +2 SD in a given population, then perhaps we can say the word is used in a value-neutral way. But that is not how 'normal' is (here I would like to say 'normally') used in ordinary or scientific language. In fact, the word has very many meanings, which are usually not specified when it is used. Table 2.2 lists various words and expressions that can replace 'normal' in everyday or scientific language.

The idea that the Gaussian distribution describes biological phenomena originated in the nineteenth century, when it was noted that the results of several anthropological measurements actually did fit quite well into the distribution. It was then inferred that there is a connection between the Gaussian function and nature: in a way nature 'wanted' organisms to have the 'right values' (Gräsbeck 1995). Vácha (1982) saw a direct connection here to Platonic thinking and an eternal idea of man. As a matter of fact, Vácha suggested that we should abandon the use of the word normal completely and replace it with other expressions.

The application of statistical normality to biomedicine has many weaknesses. The distribution of several biological phenomena is not normal: it may be skewed, it may have several peaks, it may be *lognormal* (i.e. the distribution of the logarithms of the observed values is normal), and the like. If a series of independent measurements is performed on a person, the probability of obtaining results that are outside the normal range (+2 SD) increases rapidly. After 20 tests there is a 64 % probability of 'pathological' results in at least one test (Gräsbeck 1995).

Even in the context of the geographic metaphor the authorities on IQ testing have different opinions concerning the nature of the phenomenon they are measuring.

Some of them have proposed an operational definition: intelligence is what IQ tests measure. This definition was first suggested by Boring in 1923 (Sternberg 1990) and adopted, for example, by Jensen in 1969 (Sternberg 1990). Boring did not believe in putting an end to the discussion by this circular definition; instead he saw it as a narrow definition, to be used until further scientific research allows it to be extended (Sternberg 1990).

An operational definition is, of course, problematic since there is no *gold standard* of intelligence against which the test results can be compared. Usually (e.g. in medicine), when a new diagnostic test is developed, its sensitivity and specificity are determined and expressed with reference to a gold standard.

Block and Dworkin (1974) discuss an analogy that shows the problem with operational definition. If we define temperature as what thermometers measure, we come to absurdities. We could then say that thermometers cannot be improved or that no other device can measure temperature more accurately. The early thermometers not only measured temperature but also many other things, like air pressure. IQ tests may well measure things other than intelligence, whatever intelligence is.

If there is no gold standard for developing IQ tests, what has been used as a reference? Results of IQ tests obviously correlate to *something*. They do, in fact correlate to very many things: '. . . the IQ has more correlates than any other known measurement' (Zigler *et al.* 1984, p. 225). The causal relations in the correlations are, however, complex and vague.

One of the things IQ tests correlate with is *success*. It has been argued, in fact, that a major factor involved in selecting test items is their correlation with success (Block and Dworkin 1974). The same authors argue also that these correlations are built into the tests.

The idea of measuring IQ and defining a group of people as 'intellectually disabled' is in fact value laden from the very beginning. As noted earlier, Binet's purpose was to benefit the children at the lower end of the IQ distribution. On the other hand, the values of some people may suggest that the group should be eliminated.

The definition of the American Academy of Mental Retardation

The inadequacy of the IQ-based definition has led to attempts to define ID in terms of IQ *and* some other qualities, like adaptation. One influential tradition is represented by the American Academy of Mental Retardation (AAMR).

The AAMR was founded in 1876, and, since 1921, it has published ten editions of a manual on the definition of mental retardation (MR). The fifth edition, published in 1959, brought two dramatic changes: it introduced formally the adaptive behaviour criterion to the definition and it raised the cut-off point of MR from -2 SD to -1 SD. The latter change was then overturned in the next edition in 1973.

The latest edition of the manual was published in 2002 (www.aamr.org/Policies/ faq_mental_retardation.shtml). It acknowledges the shortcomings of the term *mental retardation* but retains it. The AAMR defines MR as follows:

Definition 2

Mental retardation is a disability characterized by significant limitations both in intellectual functioning and in adaptive behavior as expressed in conceptual, social, and practical adaptive skills.

This disability originates before age 18.

Five Assumptions Essential to the Application of the Definition:

1 Limitations in present functioning must be considered within the context of community environments typical of the individual's age peers and culture.
2 Valid assessment considers cultural and linguistic diversity as well as differences in communication, sensory, motor, and behavioral factors.
3 Within an individual, limitations often coexist with strengths.
4 An important purpose of describing limitations is to develop a profile of needed supports.
5 With appropriate personalized supports over a sustained period, the life functioning of the person with mental retardation generally will improve.

The intent of the latest AAMR definitions has not been to change who is or who is not considered to have ID. Instead, the intent was to change how people *think* about ID (i.e. the emphasis shifted from the *deficiencies* of the individual to the *support* needed by the individual). In addition, the importance of the interaction between the individual and his or her environment has been stressed.

If a definition based solely on IQ (like Definition 1) is compared with the new AAMR concept, the advantages of the latter from an individual's point of view are obvious. The AAMR definition is rich and flexible, while the former is narrow and rigid. On the other hand, the latter is unsuitable, for example, for international comparisons on the prevalence of ID.

Intellectual disability and health

It is common to refer to intellectually disabled people as *not healthy* or *handicapped*. When these expressions are used, the definition is usually not given or even thought about. In the background, however, is some theory of health, disability or handicap, though it may be hidden. In the following discussion, I briefly review ID in light of two different theories of health.

Boorse's biostatistical theory of health

The first theory of health has been called the *biostatistical theory*. It is represented, for example, by the American philosopher Christopher Boorse (Boorse 1975). Boorse remarks in the beginning of his paper that we should 'distinguish sharply between theoretical health, the absence of disease and practical health', the last being a less-demanding ideal (Boorse 1975, p. 542). His goal was to analyse health and disease 'as understood by traditional physiological medicine', which he takes for granted and does not define. In the mid 1970s when Boorse's paper was written, a discussion on the nature of medicine was also launched by Engel in a famous paper criticising the so-called biomedical model (Engel 1977).

The definition Boorse proposed includes the following points (p. 562):

1 The *reference class* is a natural class of organisms of uniform functional design; specifically, an age group of a sex of a species.
2 A *normal function* of a part or process within members of the reference class is a statistically typical contribution by it to their individual survival and reproduction.
3 *Health* in a member of the reference class is *normal functional ability*: the readiness of each internal part to perform all its normal functions on typical occasions with at least typical efficiency.
4 A *disease* is a type of internal state which impairs health, i.e. reduces one or more functional abilities below typical efficiency.

Thus Boorse sees diseases as deviations from the species' biological design and their recognition as a matter of natural science, rather than as evaluative decisions.

Boorse includes both somatic and mental health in his definition, and he also mentions ID (in fact, mental retardation) on several occasions (Boorse 1975, pp. 560, 564). For him ID is an example of an *extremal disease*, which is one-sided in the sense that the other extreme (very high intelligence) is not considered a disease.

Boorse's biostatistical theory of health resembles IQ-based definitions of ID to a great degree. He refers directly to the concept of statistical distribution when he mentions ID and he also refers several times to the concept of *normal* (e.g. normal function or normal functional ability). By normal he means a statistically defined phenomenon.

Boorse seems to consider the intellectually disabled as a homogeneous group, the members of which cannot, from his point of view, be healthy. His reference class, 'an age group of a sex of a species', is a strictly biological concept, and the contribution of the relation between the individual and the external world to health or disease is ignored. Boorse does not discuss the concept of intelligence, but the way he describes mental phenomena in general suggests that his theory resembles those mentioned under the geographic and biological metaphors of mind (see the preceding discussion).

As has already been noted, the intellectually disabled are far from a homogeneous group. Even the basic distinction between the minus variants and those with organic damage (see the preceding discussion) shows that the Boorsean view is too narrow to describe ID. While it is true that many individuals with ID that is based on organic damage are not healthy according to Boorse's definition, the opposite can be said of many or most of the minus variants. The functions related to individual survival and reproduction are intact even though success in school or work may not be so.

Nordenfelt's welfare theory of health

The second theory of health has been presented by Lennart Nordenfelt in his book *On the Nature of Health* (1987). As Boorse, he aims to cover both somatic and mental health in his definition, which is based on action theory.

Nordenfelt divides theories of health into the following two categories: analytic and holistic. He criticises the former and especially Boorse's biostatistical theory. One of the main points in this critique is the inability of biostatistical theory to consider the interaction between an organism and its environment.

Nordenfelt himself promotes a holistic perspective, which he calls the *welfare theory* of health. He focuses on a person as a whole and asks whether this whole person is healthy or not. After a careful and lengthy analysis of some of his basic concepts he defines: '*A* is healthy if, and only if, *A* is able, given standard circumstances in his environment, to fulfil those goals which are necessary and jointly sufficient for his minimal happiness' (Nordenfelt 1987, p. 79).

Questions like 'what is real happiness' or 'what is minimal degree of happiness' are not scientific questions but evaluative ones in the welfare theory. These evaluations do not simply appear from nowhere; they are formed in social settings.

Nordenfelt also takes ID as an example when he discusses his welfare theory. A person with very low intelligence and a low degree of vitality sets very few and primitive goals. He is then able to fulfil these goals, and the situation permits their fulfilment. It is, however, possible that his happiness does not meet the requirements of minimal *human* happiness as it is generally understood in society.

As earlier described, we come to the division between severe and mild ID. A person with severe ID is very probably unable to fulfil his goals 'given standard circumstances in his environment'; another person with mild ID may very well be able to do so.

Concluding remarks

A comprehensive definition of ID that would cover every individual and would be suitable for all purposes does not exist, and it may not even be worth aiming at. The difference between mild and profound ID is enormous. There are no common behavioural patterns and even within one clearly defined category (like Down or fragile X syndrome) individual differences can be great (Boddington and

Podpadec 1991). The AAMR definition does not mention values or norms explicitly but admits implicitly the normative nature of the definition. The attempts to base the definition solely on IQ have also been attempts to reach a value-neutral solution, but they fail, as we have seen.

ID is clearly a normative concept, and to a large extent it has been socially constructed. Boddington and Podpadec even argue that 'what holds the class together is the assumption that they are excluded absolutely or in degree from certain valuable aspects of life' (Boddington and Podpadec, p. 183). To illustrate their conclusion they quote, for example, the discussion concerning surgery in the case of a Down syndrome child and a 'normal' child in Kuhse and Singer's *Should the Baby Live?* (1985). The authors argue that 'Down's syndrome is surely relevant to the decision to operate because it means a reduced potential for a life with the unique features which are commonly and reasonably regarded as giving special value to human lives' (Kuhse and Singer 1985, p. 140). The degree of this 'reduced potential' is not entirely dependent upon the child but is also socially conditioned (Boddington and Podpadec 1991).

In this book the concept of ID is used in two ways. When individual cases are discussed, the concept is used in the broader sense, like in the AAMR definition. However, when quantitative aspects in epidemiology and the prevention of ID are discussed, then the concept is understood in the narrower, IQ-based sense.

I have dealt with the issues of definition at length because they are so complex and because they provide the necessary background for further discussions on epidemiology and prevention.

Epidemiology of intellectual disability

Epidemiology can be defined as 'the study of the distribution and determinants of disease frequency' (Hennekens and Buring 1987, p. 3). Although the word 'disease' occurs in the definition, epidemiology deals as well with, for example, impairments and handicaps, or in the current case, ID. Originally, the term epidemiology was used almost exclusively in the context of epidemics of infectious diseases, but the changing pattern of human morbidity and mortality expanded the scope to cover all kinds of diseases, impairments and handicaps.

Disease frequency refers to the quantification of the phenomenon, and it is most frequently expressed as incidence or prevalence. Incidence quantifies the number of new events or cases of the phenomenon in a population during a specified time interval. Prevalence quantifies the proportion of individuals in a population which has the disease at a specific instant. Incidence and prevalence are interrelated, and this interrelation can be expressed mathematically by saying that prevalence (P) is proportional to the product of the incidence rate (I) and the average duration (D) of the disease as follows:

$$P = I \times D$$

Distribution of the disease considers such questions as who gets the disease, when they get it and where. Descriptive studies provide data for such practical purposes as planning health care. They are needed also for formulating hypotheses concerning possible causal or preventive factors. The term *determinant* in the definition refers to these causal factors.

Research strategies in the epidemiology of intellectual disability

The starting point of an epidemiological study is the definition of the entity to be studied. With the discussion in Chapter 2 in mind, it can be noted immediately that research on the epidemiology of ID has a major difficulty even in the very beginning. Such difficulties are not, however, unique to epidemiology. On many other occasions, too, many definitions and studies on a particular topic (e.g. bronchial asthma) are not comparable because of the lack of a common definition.

Three classical research strategies are possible, all of which have their advantages and disadvantages. These strategies are cohort (register-based), cross-sectional and case-control studies. I shall discuss each of them in light of an example.

Cohort studies

In a cohort study subjects are classified on the basis of the presence or absence of exposure to a particular factor and followed for a specified period of time to determine the development of disease in each exposure group (Hennekens and Buring 1987, p. 22). In cohort studies multiple effects of a single exposure can be examined, as can the effect of rare exposures (depending on the sample size). Prospective cohort studies with large sample sizes are, however, time consuming and expensive.

The process of identifying the intellectually disabled subjects in a population is of crucial importance to the validity of the results. Differences in the process are a major cause of the great variance in prevalence figures.

A common means of identifying intellectually disabled subjects is administrative. Persons who have been put in this category by some authority, usually medical, social or educational, are included. In such studies high prevalence figures are obtained for school years and much lower figures are found for adulthood, due to the fact that, in adulthood, adaptive behaviour takes precedence over IQ as a means of identifying ID (Richardson and Koller 1985). For the preschool years the prevalence is low because mild cases, which form the majority, are not recognised until the child attends school.

An example of a large and well-constructed cohort study on ID (and various other phenomena) is that done in two provinces in northern Finland (Rantakallio and von Wendt 1986). The study population consisted of 12 058 live births and covered 96% of all births in the region in 1966. Follow-up data were collected at various ages and a large study on ID was conducted in 1980–1981. Of the original population, 278 liveborn children had died, and only 14 could not be traced at the age of 14 years.

Information on intellectually disabled children was obtained by collecting all existing protocols for intelligence tests from health care and social welfare authorities and institutions for intellectually disabled children. A special inquiry concerning all children not attending school at a level appropriate for their age was also made.

The prevalence of ID at the age of 14 years was 11.9 per 1000, and the prevalence of intellectual subnormality (IQ 71 to 85) was 13.7 per 1000. The authors noted that they had obtained higher prevalence figures, especially for severe ID, than most earlier studies, and they discussed the possible explanations at length.

They suggested that the difference could be partially explained by the exceptionally successful follow-up (only 1.2 per 1000 children could not be traced at 14 years of age).

It is worth noting that the definition of ID in this survey was based solely on IQ measurements.

Cross-sectional studies

A cross-sectional study is a survey in which a population is not followed-up over time but is instead assessed at a particular point of time. In a way, a cross-sectional survey provides a 'snapshot' of the health status of the population (Hennekens and Buring 1987).

An example of a cross-sectional survey on ID is a project conducted in the Kuopio province in Finland (Kääriäinen *et al.* 1985). Four birth cohorts born in 1969–1972 were screened in two phases, first at school followed by those who scored low being given psychological tests. Altogether 12 882 children were screened, and the prevalence for ID was 13.8 per 1000. The research project was multi-disciplinary, and several reports concerning the medical, dental, social and economic aspects of ID were produced.

One of the most interesting findings in the Kuopio project was that, of the mildly intellectually disabled, 81% and, of the severely intellectually disabled children, 18% were unregistered and therefore outside special services. This fact, of course, reflects partly the supply of these services, but it also reveals how unreliable the administrative criterion may be in the assessment of ID.

Case-control studies

In a case-control study subjects are selected on the basis of whether they do (cases) or do not (controls) have the particular disease under study (Hennekens and Buring 1987). The groups are then compared with respect to a characteristic or an exposure. The case-control strategy is useful in the evaluation of rare diseases, and it allows the study of diseases with very long latency periods. On the other hand, this strategy does not allow direct computation of incidence or prevalence rates. The selection of cases and controls must be done with extreme care, and the setting is still prone to bias.

Case-control studies can evaluate a wide range of potential aetiologic factors, and they are therefore used to test specific hypotheses or create new hypotheses concerning aetiology.

An example of a case-control study on ID is the survey done by Louhiala (1993) in an area in southern and central Finland. The identification of the relevant cases was made mainly on the basis of the registers of three districts of special care for the intellectually disabled. Perinatal data concerning 33 factors possibly associated with risk for ID were then collected from the 12 maternity hospitals in the area. One control for each case was randomly selected from the hospital delivery book covering the birth year of the case child.

Independent risk indicators for ID were low maternal social class, multiparity, multiple pregnancy, male sex, small for gestational age, asphyxia, hypoglycaemia and hyperbilirubinaemia in the newborn. The risk for ID in association with a low Apgar score and very low birthweight (<1500 g) seemed to increase, while the risk associated with moderately low birthweight seemed to decrease in the 1970s, when neonatal intensive care was introduced. This finding was not surprising, because the tiniest babies usually died before the introduction of intensive care, and there was no possibility for them to become disabled.

Prevalence of intellectual disability

Of the two commonest measures in epidemiology, incidence and prevalence, the former is not useful in ID research, as it would require the possibility to determine the intellectual status of newborn babies, which is not feasible, if intelligence is understood as it is operationalised in present IQ tests. The concepts of intelligence and ID can be applied only to older children, and especially mild ID is often noticed as late as school age. Therefore, the occurrence of ID is commonly expressed in terms of prevalence figures.

The variation in the methodological strategies used and the probable true differences between populations explain the wide range of prevalence rates, between 9 and 80 per 1000 children (Richardson and Koller 1985). The figures obtained for severe ID are more stable than those for mild ID. Tables 3.1 and 3.2 show some prevalence figures from various parts of the world. The huge differences between those for Maine and Salford and, on the other hand, between age groups illustrate the influence of methodology and also the difficulties of comparative epidemiology in this area.

Abramowicz and Richardson (1975) reviewed 27 epidemiological studies of severe ID and concluded that a remarkable consistency existed in the prevalence, approximating 4 per 1000. They wrote:

The best approximation of the 'true' prevalence rate of severe mental retardation appears to be between 3 to 5 per 1000. For those reliable studies that present prevalence rates for older children, the median 'true' prevalence of severe mental retardation is 3.7 per 1000 and the average 'true' prevalence is 3.96 per 1000. Since cases of severe mental retardation in a community can be missed and because there may be a tendency to overestimate a child's potential by classifying him as mildly rather that severely mentally retarded, the average figure of 4 per 1000 age-specific population is probably a fair estimate of the number of severely retarded children who require services in a community. (Abramowicz and Richardson 1975, p. 29)

Table 3.1. Prevalence figures for severe intellectual disability[*]

Year	Place	Age group (years)	Prevalence (per 1000)	Notes
1960	London	10–14	2.8	
1966	Amsterdam	10–14	5.2	Administrative assessment
		10 and 15	7.3	Individual assessment
1970	Aarhus	10–14	4.5	
1980	N. Finland	14	6.4	
1982	Kuopio	10–11	6.3	

Table 3.2. Prevalence figures for mild intellectual disability[*]

Year	Place	Age group (years)	Prevalence (per 1000)	Notes
1957	Maine	5–9	16.3	Predominantly rural, lower
		10–14	35.1	socio-economic class, upper
		15–19	16.1	IQ limit 75
1961	Salford	5–9	0.4	
		10–14	0.3	
		15–19	8.7	
1966	Amsterdam	10	14.3	
1980	N. Finland	14	5.5	
1982	Kuopio	10–11	6.3	

[*]Data adapted from Richardson and Koller 1985, Kääriäinen 1985 and Rantakallio and von Wendt 1986

Fryers (1984) has strongly criticised the way prevalence rates are assumed to be stable and the way temporal and geographic variations are ignored. It is worth noting that Abramowicz and Richardson (1975) discuss 'true', not true prevalence, and they present 4 per 1000 as a fair estimate of severely intellectually disabled children who require services in the community. In fact, in the studies they found reliable, the prevalence varied between 2.6 and 5.5 per 1000.

Causes of intellectual disability

If the definition (or part of the definition) of a phenomenon refers to a statistical distribution (like the normal distribution), speaking of causes of that phenomenon is not always sensible. At the population level it is obvious that part of the population

Table 3.3. Classification of disorders in which intellectual disability can occur and examples for each category

Class	Examples
1. Preconceptional	
1.1. Chromosomal causes	Down syndrome (trisomy 21)
1.2. X-linked causes	Fragile X syndrome
1.3. Other genetic causes	Phenylketonuria (PKU)
2. Prenatal	
2.1. Malformations of the central nervous system	Anencephaly, spina bifida, hydrocephalus, microcephaly
2.2. Malformation syndromes	
2.3. Environmental causes	Foetal alcohol syndrome (FAS), cocaine-induced brain damage, irradiation during pregnancy
3. Perinatal	
3.1. Intrauterine disorders	Placental insufficiency, obstetrical trauma
3.2. Neonatal disorders	Hypoxic-ischaemic encephalopathy, intra-ventricular haemorrhage, infection, hypoglycaemia
4. Postnatal	
4.1. Head injuries	Cerebral contusion
4.2. Infections	Meningitis
4.3. Psychosocial causes	
4.4. Other causes	Cerebral anoxia (e.g. near-drowning)
5. Unknown causes	

is necessarily present and meets the criterion. At the individual level, on the other hand, it may be impossible to conclude whether a person is disabled plainly because he happens to be at the 'wrong end' of the distribution or whether methods are merely lacking for determining the cause.

In cases in which a causal factor can be determined, the factor cannot, however, be proclaimed as the 'ultimate cause', since causality is a complex phenomenon and involves a chain or web of different causal agents. Even for Down syndrome the ultimate cause is unknown, although for many purposes it is sufficient to say that an extra chromosome 21 is responsible.

In the following discussion the concept of cause should be considered as a practical term that expresses current knowledge of the essential part or item of the causal chain leading to ID. Table 3.3 presents a classification of disorders that lead to severe or mild ID and also some examples. More comprehensive lists are available in, for example, Fryers' work (1984) and in the AAMR manual (American Association on Mental Retardation 1992).

The classification in Table 3.3 is based on the timing of the primary event. In many cases the timing is, however, difficult or impossible to determine. An increased understanding of the underlying pathological mechanisms may influence the location of a disorder in the classification. The commonest change occurs when a single genetic defect is found in a disorder, which so far has been placed in categories 2.2 or 5. Multiple locations are also possible for many entities (e.g. microcephaly may be of genetic origin or it may originate during pregnancy). Category 4.3 is problematic in the sense that, in many cases, it is impossible to determine whether ID is a result of the influence of genes or due to adverse environmental conditions during infancy and childhood. The latter is mentioned in most classifications, but its nature is seldom specified. Kurtz (1977, p. 52) suggests that

... products of an aberrant subculture are not mentally retarded in the sense that they do not possess the biological capacity to perform in an acceptable manner; rather, the subcultures which are significant to them have emphasised behaviours that are not sampled by intelligence tests – i.e., they may have 'correctly' learned the 'wrong' things.

Other forms of classifications are possible and feasible; for instance Fryers has used the main classes of primary disorders (present at conception, like Down syndrome), primary disorders with secondary neurologic sequelae as a secondary effect, like phenylketonuria (PKU), and secondary disorders, like foetal alcohol syndrome (FAS).

Trends in the epidemiology of intellectual disability

Very few studies have been reported on changes in the occurrence of ID. This lack is understandable because the methodological difficulties are obvious. Administrative definitions of ID are very much related to the resources available, and therefore analyses of time trends are not feasible. Cross-sectional studies done at certain intervals could be useful, but, due to the small prevalence rates, such studies are expensive and laborious. The validity of a comparison in which the same IQ tests have been administered to age cohorts between, for example, 10- or 20-year intervals, can also be questioned.

Changes over time in the same population were studied in Salford, England, between 1951 and 1980 (Fryers 1984). The object of the study was severe ID (IQ < 50) and the case finding was based on existing registers. The prevalence for the age group of 5 to 9 years increased through the 1960s and early 1970s from 1.89 to 5.07 and decreased thereafter to 3.57 in 1980.

As reasons for the increase in prevalence, Fryers mentioned improved case finding, a general increase in survival and differential migration, by which he meant that families with intellectually impaired children elect to move to the area (known for good services) more often than did other families.

The reasons for the decrease in prevalence in the next decade are less obvious. Fryers suggested that a reduced incidence of some specific syndromes like PKU and kernicterus due to blood group incompatibility was at least possible.

It may be that it is not sensible to speculate about the overall changes in the prevalence of ID *in general*. The focus could be on specific groups, like the most severely disabled who require many services. There is also a need to follow the occurrence of specific disorders as a part of the quality control of health care in general and preventive measures in particular.

One indirect method for studying time trends is to survey risk factors and changes in them over time. There is, for instance, some evidence that the risk for ID associated with a low Apgar score increased after the introduction of modern neonatal intensive care (Louhiala 1993). It was assumed that, earlier, babies with low scores very often died and the survivors did not carry a significant risk for ID, but with intensive care more babies with severe brain damage survive.

Some data concerning changes in the prevalence of ID can also be obtained in the context of research on other handicaps. The epidemiology of cerebral palsy (CP) is much easier to study and data from England suggest that the prevalence of severe ID in association with CP slightly increased during the 1980s (Nicholson and Alberman 1992).

4

Prevention of intellectual disability: general issues

'It is better to be healthy than ill or dead. That is the beginning and the end of the only real argument for preventive medicine. It is sufficient.' These lines were written by Geoffrey Rose in his book *The Strategy of Preventive Medicine* (Rose 1992, p. 4), which is an introduction to the ideas behind preventive medicine at the individual and population levels. The citation is the *humanitarian argument* for prevention. Rose also described the *economic argument*, which, according to him, proves to be misleading or even false when scrutinised more closely in individual cases.

Rose writes about preventive medicine, which, of course, covers intellectual disability only partly. As seen in Chapter 2, ID is not exclusively (and in many cases not at all) a medical matter but is also a social construction. Thus a person with ID may be healthy and the discussion about prevention must go beyond the scope of medicine. In this chapter the concept of prevention is first defined. Secondly, the question '*Why* should ID be prevented?' is introduced. Thirdly, the general strategies and practical possibilities for preventing ID are described. Fourthly, the ethical issues that arise in the context of this prevention are briefly introduced.

Levels of prevention

Prevention is usually divided into three levels: primary, secondary and tertiary (American Association on Mental Retardation 1992).

Primary prevention refers to actions that occur before the onset of the problem and that stop the problem from occurring. *Secondary prevention* refers to actions that shorten the duration of, or reverse the effects of, existing problems. *Tertiary prevention* refers to actions that limit the adverse consequences of a problem and improve the individual's level of functioning.

It is obvious that preventive activities concerning ID may be both medical and social, behavioural or educational. Examples of primary prevention are vaccination against *Haemophilus influenzae* type B meningitis (medical), prenatal care, support to avoid FAS (behavioural/educational) and general welfare programmes (social). Examples of the secondary prevention of ID are newborn screening of PKU (medical) and early infant intervention in high-risk families (educational). Tertiary prevention concentrates on people with ID in the form of, for example, optimised medical care (e.g. regular screening for hypothyreosis in Down syndrome) and various educational programmes.

On many occasions, the primary prevention of ID means the same as the prevention of the medical condition leading to ID, and the ethical problems are thus equivalent. There is, however, a form of primary prevention of ID that differs from the usual methods of preventing disease or disability. This radically different method, which has a unique spectrum of ethical problems, is the prevention of the *existence* of the people or persons with the probability to become intellectually disabled at some stage in life.

Why should intellectual disability be prevented?

The first and crucial question with respect to the prevention of ID is, of course, *why* should it be prevented? Later in this book a long chapter (Chapter 7) will be devoted to a thorough discussion of this topic. At this stage, however, it is necessary to describe briefly the main points. Although there are various and extensive prevention programmes (like serum screening for Down syndrome), this question has not been widely discussed. Instead it has been taken for granted that prevention per se is a good thing.

The primary aim of the prevention of a disease or a handicap is usually to help the person who is thought to suffer from the disease or handicap in question. As regards ID, the situation is different. Of course there can be strategies that are successful in preventing both painful and deadly diseases *and* ID (like vaccination against *Haemophilus influenzae* type B infection). On a general level, however, it is not only the well-being of the (future) intellectually disabled person that is at issue, but also the well-being of the family and society.

The reasons for wanting to prevent ID are to avoid negative consequences in the following areas:
- economic impact on families
- economic impact on society
- disruption of families
- quality of life of persons with ID.

Each of these areas has been dealt with in detail in Chapter 7, but some preliminary remarks nevertheless follow.

There is anecdotal evidence of the economic burden that an intellectually disabled child causes to his or her family. However, little systematic empirical research has been done on this topic. At least in developed societies the possible additional costs are, to a great extent, borne by society or, for example, insurance companies.

There are also few exact data on the economic burden placed on society by intellectually disabled people. It is obvious that a person who, for instance, is never able to work increases the burden. On the other hand, there are programmes and legislation that try to enable persons with handicaps to function like other people, be employed and become self-sufficient. The recent trend to close massive institutions and integrate the disabled into society probably also decreases the economic burden on society.

An intellectually disabled child always brings about a crisis in a family, but the impact is not entirely negative. There are both families that have been weakened and families that report to have been enriched by the presence of a disabled child.

Anyone who has had some contact with intellectually disabled people can relate anecdotes about happy and social individuals with ID whose quality of life is obviously high, or, on the other hand, they know of intellectually disabled individuals with severe physical handicaps who seem to suffer greatly through much of their lives. It should, however, be recognised that the experience of persons with ID may be very different from that of the people who know them. The few studies that have been done on the quality of life of intellectually disabled people provide mixed evidence, and it is not clear whether the ones who are unhappy feel bad because they are disabled or because they have been poorly cared for (Rose-Ackerman 1982).

Attitudes towards intellectual disability

It is often useful to take a brief look at history to obtain a wider view of a phenomenon. Since attitudes towards ID have varied greatly, I shall give a short overview of them in both Western societies and some other cultures.

In ancient Rome and Greece, the intellectually disabled were treated as objects of scorn and persecution. Early Christianity brought some pity for the intellectually disabled as St Paul had asked to 'comfort the feeble-minded'. In medieval times they served as fools or jesters or were regarded as 'les enfants du Bon Dieu', who were wandering about the streets of Europe (Rosen *et al.* 1976). An abnormal child could also be thought to be a 'changeling', a child of nature demons of semihuman form (Boddington and Podpadec 1991). In England, the distinction between the born fool and the lunatic was made for the first time in the thirteenth century.

Superstition still prevailed during the Reformation when both Luther and Calvin regarded the intellectually disabled as 'filled with Satan' (Rosen *et al.* 1976). The revitalised interest in education and humanitarianism during the Renaissance may have paved the way for the educational movement of the nineteenth century.

The nineteenth century brought about many changes, both in the lives of the disabled and also in the attitudes of other people. The first special schools were founded both in Europe and in the United States and, beginning about 1866, 'idiocy' ceased being regarded as a unitary and homogeneous condition (Rosen *et al.* 1976). The changes in the goals of those dealing with the intellectually disabled were rapid. First came the desire to 'make the deviant undeviant' (between 1850 and 1880), then to shelter 'the deviant from society' (1870 to 1890) and finally to protect 'society from the deviant' (1880 to 1900) (White and Wolfensberger 1969, cited by Rosen *et al.* 1976, p. xix).

At the turn of the twentieth century attitudes towards the intellectually disabled had gradually changed, and such people were often regarded as a menace (Rosen *et al.* 1976). The popularisation of the works of Darwin and Mendel inspired studies on human heredity, which carried an aura of science. Richard Dugdale, for example, studied the Juke family over seven generations and found a large number of prostitutes, deformed persons, paupers, criminals, and lazy, weak-minded and blind individuals but only one case of idiocy (Dugdale 1877, reprinted in Rosen *et al.* 1976). It is surprising how Dugdale's own interpretation of poor environmental conditions leading to degeneracy in this family was replaced later by the conclusion that heredity was the main factor and that actually half of the family had been feebleminded.

During the same years the population with ID appeared to be scientifically identifiable by the use of standardised intelligence tests that had recently been developed in France. An influential American scientist, Henry Goddard, who had translated and popularised Binet's work, was convinced that feeblemindedness was hereditary and that the intellectual capacity of an individual was irreversible. Goddard described another family, the Kallikaks, for whom he identified 480 descendants of a feebleminded girl. Only 46 of these were normal, others were feebleminded, illegitimate, sexually immoral, alcoholic, epileptic or criminal (Bourguignon 1994).

Goddard and his followers started the eugenics movement, which argued for the segregation of the disabled from society, sterilisation as a means of alleviating the problem of the spread of feeblemindedness in society, restrictions on the immigration of undesirable classes, and marriage restrictions for the feebleminded, the epileptic, the criminal and others.

An article by a prominent representative of the eugenics movement, Reverend Karl Schwartz, illustrates the spirit of it (Schwartz 1908). He began by stating that 'it is not a pessimistic view of life to wish to see a man get out of the world, who is not fit for it, and who has little or no chance of ever becoming so' (Schwartz 1908, p. 149). By the unfit he did not mean only profoundly intellectually and physically handicapped individuals but 'an idle, inefficient and vicious class' that would 'sap the strength of the strong' (Schwartz, p. 149).

Schwartz further wrote that 'abnormal individuals are not only valueless but are generally harmful to society; for besides being nonproducers, they absorb the energies and the productive power of others. Hence, in the development of a people it becomes necessary that the lifetime of these abnormal individuals should be shortened' (Schwartz, p. 150).

The eugenics movement in America never widely adopted this extreme position but, for instance, compulsory sterilisation remained a common practice for decades.

In Germany, however, the direct medical killing of defective individuals who would harm the *volk* was proposed in the 1920s and became the practice a decade later. Falsified medical records were kept to create the impression that doctors sought to cure rather than kill defective children (Bourguignon 1994). The age of the children involved gradually moved upwards and also individuals with minor impairments, juvenile delinquents and eventually Jews were drawn into the euthanasia project.

The eugenics movement gradually lost its scientific backing during the first decades of the twentieth century as intelligence research began to show that intelligence is modifiable (Skeels and Dye 1939), and increasing knowledge showed that not all the causes behind ID were genetic (Rosen *et al.* 1976).

Major changes in the attitudes towards the intellectually disabled occurred during World War II. Manpower needs were severe and mildly disabled men were released from institutions for the armed forces or defence work in factories. The success of these men was one starting point for the de-institutionalisation movement of later decades (Rosen *et al.* 1976).

The development in the attitudes toward intellectually disabled people after the war has been described in terms of the 'normalisation' principle. Normalisation means that the living environment of the disabled should resemble that of the non-disabled as much as possible and that they should have as independent a life as possible. De-institutionalisation has taken place as a sign of this normalisation.

Labelling

A 10-year-old boy was admitted to a child psychiatric ward after a suicide attempt. There he was found to be intellectually subnormal although he attended an ordinary primary school. He was an adopted child of parents in high academic positions who apparently had expected their only child to do well in school, and this expectation had caused frustration which gradually grew unbearable and led to the suicide attempt. Would this have happened if the intellectual subnormality of the child had been noticed earlier (i.e. is it possible that *labelling* the boy as intellectually subnormal would have given him and his family some advantage)? In general, is there any advantage for an individual, for the family or for society in having someone decide that the individual meets certain criteria for ID?

A label can be seen as 'a verbal or linguistic device that, in its most fundamental terms, creates and sustains a world' (McCullough 1984). At the same time, as the individual gains a world, he or she also loses a world (i.e. the world of the rest of us). The world gained through the label ID means entitlement to special treatment and education aimed at helping the person in question overcome or ameliorate difficulties in private and social life. The world lost means losing full moral worth as a bearer of rights and responsibilities.

Labelling individuals as intellectually disabled can be justified for the following three reasons: the benefit to the person, the benefit to society and the benefit of maintaining the integrity of observation and description (Kopelman 1984). Whatever the justification for labelling a person as intellectually disabled, something is also always lost. To be recognised as intellectually disabled may mean that one is endowed with a 'master status', which becomes a central characteristic of the individual (Kurtz 1977).

As an example of a benefit to society Kopelman mentions people who are not entitled to drive a car because they cannot understand road signs. She calls for a heavy burden of proof to demonstrate this kind of justification for labelling people. The third justification for labelling, maintaining the integrity of observation and description, cannot function alone; there cannot be a situation in which labelling a person as intellectually disabled would not benefit him or her or society but still would be important for research, for example.

Must the world gained, special education, special treatment and the like always be purchased at the price of a world lost or diminished moral status? Probably something is always lost, but the loss may not be a universal loss of rights since the two worlds are not necessarily logically connected (McCullough 1984). If we take a case-by-case view, instead of looking at the disabled as a class, it may be possible to balance the loss of rights so that it is individually tailored to meet the specific situations that will be faced in life.

General strategies for the prevention of intellectual disability

On the basis of the preceding discussion, it is obvious that there are two very different approaches to the issue of preventing ID. The first concentrates on the individual level, and the idea is to find strategies to eliminate the causes leading to the excess number of persons at the lower end of the IQ distribution. The second tries to influence the environment so that a person with subnormal intellectual functioning

Table 4.1. Examples of strategies for prevention

Aetiology	Examples
1. Preconceptional	
1.1. Chromosomal causes	Prenatal screening (e.g. for Down syndrome)
1.2. Other genetic causes	Newborn screening (e.g. for phenylketonuria)
2. Prenatal	
2.1. Malformations of the central nervous system	Folate therapy during pregnancy, ultrasound screening
2.2. Malformation syndromes	
2.3. Environmental causes	Health education (e.g. about alcohol, drugs and radiation during pregnancy)
3. Perinatal	
3.1. Intrauterine disorders	Optimal prenatal and obstetric care
3.2. Neonatal disorders	Optimal neonatal care
4. Postnatal	
4.1. Head injuries	Health education (e.g. cycling helmets)
4.2. Infections	Vaccinations, health education, optimal care

can better adapt to society and would thus not be intellectually disabled in the sense of the AAMR definition. Table 4.1 lists some examples of the former approach.

The issue of prevention can also be considered in terms of theoretical or practical possibilities. Theoretically a large proportion of severe ID (with an organic background) can be prevented. On the other hand, practical possibilities are limited.

In cases in which the aetiology of ID is entirely genetic, it would theoretically be possible to eliminate the entire category if a complete genetic map of the foetus were available and all foetuses with defective genes were aborted. Even scientifically, however, such actions are not possible in the foreseeable future, and the practical possibilities for eliminating genetically determined ID are limited.

Theoretically, it is possible to eliminate obstetrical, neonatal and paediatric complications leading to ID, but, again, the practical possibilities are limited. In fact, neonatological developments may also *increase* the number of intellectually disabled persons in the category of very low birthweight babies.

The development in medical diagnostics has decreased the number of cases in which the aetiology is unknown. Even today, however, there are many individuals whose ID probably has some somatic, but so far unknown, background. It can be expected that this category will become smaller but that it cannot be eliminated totally.

A summary of the theoretical and practical possibilities of preventing ID is presented in Table 4.2.

Table 4.2. Theoretical and practical possibilities for preventing intellectual disability. $+++$ refers to complete or nearly complete, $++$ to great and $+$ to limited preventability

Aetiology of ID	Theoretical possibilities	Practical possibilities
1. Preconceptional causes	$+++$	$+$
2. Prenatal		
2.1. Malformations of the central nervous system	$++$	$+$
2.2. Malformation syndromes	$++$	$+$
2.3. Environmental causes	$++$	$+$
3. Perinatal		
3.1. Intrauterine disorders	$++$	$+$
3.2. Neonatal disorders	$++$	$+$
4. Postnatal		
4.1. Head injuries	$++$	$+$
4.2. Infections	$++$	$+$
4.3. Psychosocial causes	$+$	
5. Unknown causes	$++$	$+$

Ethical problems in the prevention of intellectual disability: introduction

The two different approaches mentioned in the previous chapter for the prevention of ID should be kept in mind when ethical problems are considered. At the practical level, however, these strategies overlap. Actions taken towards an environment in which persons with subnormal intellectual functioning can better adapt to society can be considered primary prevention for ID in the group of the *minus variants* (see Chapter 2), but it can also be considered secondary prevention in the group of intellectually disabled people with organic brain damage.

The variety of strategies used in the prevention of ID is great. It is obvious that the range of ethical issues involved is large, from problems related to the individuals concerned to problems at the level of society as a whole. Technically, there is great variation, too, with some strategies being extremely complex and others being relatively simple. An example of a preventive strategy that is non-problematic both technically and ethically is the addition of iodine to salt in certain geographic areas to prevent hypothyreosis. A good example of a strategy that is highly problematic both technically and ethically is serum screening to prevent Down syndrome. The prevention of FAS is an example of prevention that is biologically simple (do not use alcohol during pregnancy) but ethically complex.

In the following discussion I briefly describe the ethical problems that arise in the process of prevention. They are also summarised in Table 4.3.

Table 4.3. Outline of ethical problems in the prevention of intellectual disability in various aetiological subgroups

1. Preconceptional causes
    Access to prenatal diagnosis
    Individual or societal level of prevention
    Directive or non-directive counselling
2. Prenatal causes
    Autonomy in antenatal care (e.g. foetal alcohol syndrome)
    Ethical problems related to ultrasound screening
3. Perinatal causes
    Malformed newborn: quality of life; who decides
    Newborn with brain damage: quality of life; who decides
4. Postnatal causes
    Large prevention programmes (e.g. vaccinations)
    Parental refusal of therapy

Preconception causes

Prenatal diagnostics are available today for many genetically determined diseases and conditions, also those leading to ID. Depending on the system of health care, prenatal services are offered either publicly or privately. In many countries both the private and public sectors of health care perform these diagnostics.

Another question with respect to prenatal diagnostics is the focus of the action itself. When worries about eugenics are expressed in this context, the activity is defended on the grounds that it is the women themselves and the families who are of primary concern, not society in general. Thus the primary aim would *not* be to prevent ID in general, but to help women and families to make an informed decision concerning reproduction. The situation is not so clear, however, since trends toward seeing prevention at the societal level as the primary aim also exist. The question is currently highly relevant with respect to screening for Down syndrome, and I deal with this question in detail in Chapter 5.

The nature of genetic counselling is also relevant here. It is obvious that counselling can never be value neutral, but whether value neutrality should be the aim still remains a question. This is a general issue relevant to all genetic counselling and also counselling for conditions originating later in the pre-, peri- or postnatal period.

Prenatal causes

Foetal alcohol syndrome has been mentioned as an example of a prenatal cause leading to ID. From a purely biological point of view its prevention would be very simple ('do not drink alcohol during pregnancy') but developing practices in antenatal care to prevent FAS has proved extremely challenging and also ethically problematic. The main ethical issue is about the autonomy of the pregnant woman and the possible paternalism of the health care personnel involved.

It is sometimes not possible to define the timing of the accident leading to brain damage and further to ID. Second-trimester ultrasound screening can detect such brain damage in many cases and is in practice in many countries. It is obvious that serious ethical problems are involved in the implementation of ultrasound screening.

Perinatal causes

If prenatal ultrasound screening has not been performed, or sometimes even in spite of it, a malformation may be diagnosed only after birth. Serious brain damage may also be the result of difficulties during the perinatal period itself. In both cases parents and health care personnel have to face serious ethical issues such as who should decide about the possible withdrawal of life support or whose quality of life is at stake.

Postnatal causes

As shown in the previous chapters, only a minor part of ID with an organic background originates after the perinatal period. The major causes during this period are various diseases and accidents leading to brain damage. Some of these diseases (like meningitis caused by *Meningococcus* or *Haemophilus influenzae* type B) can be prevented by vaccinations, and parental refusal of such vaccinations may be the ultimate cause of ID in the individual. Similarly, for religious or other reasons, parents may deny their child therapy for such a disease and thus put him or her at risk of death or permanent injury.

Concluding remarks

The prevention of ID can take place at many levels, and only some of these levels involve medical activities. Primary prevention is sometimes possible, but secondary or tertiary prevention is no less important. All forms of prevention may be ethically and technically simple or complex. Even the question 'why should ID be prevented' does not have a simple answer.

In the following chapters, I focus on ethical issues that arise in the context of the prevention of ID due to preconception causes. Ethical issues arising with respect to the other groups are, however, often similar. Parental autonomy and the roles of society and the medical community are examples of such questions.

5

Prenatal diagnosis and screening

During the past four decades several techniques have been developed to enable physicians and geneticists to estimate the risk for certain diseases, syndromes and conditions or to set the exact diagnosis already during the foetal period. On the other hand, effective possibilities for curing or preventing these conditions have not been developed as rapidly. In fact, only foetal transfusions to manage, for example, serious blood group incompatibility can be considered routine treatment. Other forms of foetal therapy are still experimental.

One of the justifications for developing these new techniques has been that, in the future, it would be possible to treat conditions that we first learn to assess. One of the major rationalisations given to the human genome project has been that the characterisation of the human genome would lead to therapeutic innovations.

Prenatal investigations can be in the form of either *screening* or *diagnostics*. These terms are not used consistently, and they overlap, but in general the results of screening may be the demonstration of an increased risk for a certain condition (like Down syndrome or neural tube defect) or a definitive diagnosis. In a diagnostic procedure a definitive diagnosis is obtained or excluded, within the limits of uncertainty allowed by the chosen method. While, in the health care context in general, people come to ask for help, screening investigations are offered to people without any symptoms. An example of a test that can perform both a screening and a diagnostic function is ultrasonography.

In screening 'a population group is examined with the aim of mapping the occurrence of a particular trait; in some cases, this includes tracing those people who have the trait concerned' (The Danish Council of Ethics 1993, p. 47). Health screening has its origins in the nineteenth century ideas about regular precautionary medical examinations for adults. Early in the twentieth century an analogy with the regular check-ups needed for automobiles was presented (Nelkin and Tancredi 1995). Interest in preventive medicine declined in the 1920s and 1930s but increased again after World War II (Nelkin and Trancredi 1995).

Genetic screening in general means the study of the occurrence of persons with a specific gene or chromosome composition in a population (The Danish Council of Ethics 1993). The first widespread screening test was for the detection of PKU in newborns. Untreated PKU leads to intellectual disability, but, with a modified diet from birth on, normal intellectual development can be accomplished.

In the guidelines of the World Health Organization, the following requirements have been given for screening programmes (Nelkin and Trancredi 1995, p. 68):

1 The disease must constitute a major health problem.
2 There must be an accepted treatment for patients diagnosed as having the disease.
3 Diagnostic and therapeutic facilities must be available.
4 The disease must be demonstrable in a latent or early symptomatic stage.
5 A suitable test or examination method must be available.
6 The test/examination method must be acceptable to the population.
7 The progress of the disease in untreated cases – including development from latent to manifest phases – must have been adequately clarified.
8 The treatment indications must be clearly defined.
9 The cost of detecting the disease (including diagnosis and treatment of patients) must be in reasonable proportion to the health service's total expenditure.
10 The screening action must be an ongoing process, not an on-off phenomenon.

It is easy to note that prenatal screening meets questionably some of these requirements. If the pregnant woman is considered the patient, then the 'treatment' in most cases would be abortion. If, on the other hand, the foetus is the patient, the treatment would, in most cases, mean killing the patient. The preceding list was obviously created with diseases like breast cancer or prostate cancer in mind.

These reservations have been taken into consideration in the report of the Dutch Health Council on genetic screening (Hoedemaekers 1998). It does not, for example, explicitly require that acceptable treatment must be available. Instead, it proposes that meaningful options must be available for the persons screened. Noteworthy also is the fact that the Dutch report no longer requires that the condition screened be serious.

In the following discussion the term prenatal diagnosis refers to procedures in which a definitive diagnosis for the foetus can be obtained or excluded prenatally, and prenatal screening concerns procedures that provide risk estimates for certain foetal conditions.

History

The widespread use of prenatal diagnosis is a recent phenomenon, but its history is longer than usually thought, dating back to the 1950s. (The following sketch of the history of prenatal diagnosis is based on Cowan (1994).) It seems not to be a product of deliberate research and development, but rather a side-product of basic medical research (Munthe 1996).

Separate groups of scientists in three countries discovered simultaneously that the sex of human foetuses could be predicted by analysing cells from the amniotic fluid. The first reported abortion after prenatal diagnosis through amniocentesis was performed in 1960. A diagnosis of a disease was not set, only the sex of the foetus was determined. The mother was a carrier of haemophilia, and the foetus was male, thus a possible haemophiliac had it been born. The first abortions due to the chromosomal diagnosis of Down syndrome were performed in 1968.

The first invasive technique used in prenatal diagnosis, amniocentesis, was still in a developmental phase and was applied narrowly in the early 1970s, but some non-medical events that took place at that time formed the grounds for the diffusion phase of that technology.

Firstly, in the USA, several lawsuits were settled in which parents of disabled children sued for malpractice when an obstetrician had not referred a woman over the age of 35 years for amniocentesis. Because of the success of these lawsuits, the American College of Obstetricians and Gynecologists and the American Academy of Pediatrics advised their members to offer prenatal diagnostic services or referrals for prenatal diagnosis to avoid the risk of being taken to court (Cowan 1994).

Secondly, the diffusion of amniocentesis could not have taken place without the simultaneous reformation of abortion laws in many countries (e.g. the USA, Canada and Great Britain) (Cowan 1994). It has even been argued that legalised abortion was *the* prerequisite for the development of prenatal diagnosis (Reid 1991). The changes in social values in the late 1960s and early 1970s occurred, however, simultaneously with the advent of amniocentesis, and it is not easy to determine the impact of one on the other (Reid 1991).

The development in genetics has already had a great impact on diagnostics, screening and counselling. Its impact on prevention has so far been based only on abortions that have been performed after diagnostic procedures and practically no therapeutic forms of intervention have become available. There still remains a serious gap between disease characterisation and treatment (Friedmann 1990).

The total effect of prenatal screening and diagnosis on the occurrence of the conditions searched for is difficult to estimate because of the fluctuation of the prevalences. In some cases, like Down syndrome, changes in the maternal-age profile cause changes in the prevalence. It is, however, obvious that the total effect of prenatal screening and diagnosis on the population level is small. For example, the history of the settlement of an area, immigration and family size are factors that have far greater effect on the genetic structure of a population than prenatal diagnosis, even when taken to an extreme (Simola 1995).

Methods

Amniocentesis and chorionic villus sampling are the most widely used invasive techniques in prenatal diagnosis. The former is usually performed at 15 to 16 weeks of gestation. About 20 ml of amniotic fluid is aspirated from the uterus, after location of the placenta by ultrasonography. Results are obtained within 1 to 4 weeks, depending on the nature of the test. The risk of miscarriage associated with amniocentesis is 0.5% to 1.0% (D'Alton and DeCherney 1993, Kingston 1994).

In chorionic villus sampling, foetally derived chorionic villus material is obtained transcervically with a flexible catheter between 9 and 12 weeks' gestation. The sampling is also performed under ultrasonographic guidance. The procedure increases the risk for miscarriage slightly more than amniocentesis, but the experience of the operator may be crucial for the outcome (D'Alton and DeCherney 1993). In the early 1990s a serious side effect, absent or defective limbs of the newborn, was reported after the procedure (D'Alton and DeCherney 1993). The association is not, however, clear, and a later registry-based analysis could not confirm the association (Froster and Jackson 1996).

A rarer invasive technique is foetoscopy, which is performed during the second trimester in cases in which the foetus must be seen directly to identify dysmorphic features or to obtain foetal samples (Kingston 1994).

A non-invasive method of prenatal diagnosis is ultrasonography, which in its original one-dimensional mode enabled the diagnosis of hydrocephalus in the 1970s. The technique has developed rapidly, and today the detection of, for example, clefts of the lip and palate, as well as structural abnormalities of the brain and heart, is possible (Kingston 1994).

In the future it may also be possible to ascertain the karyotype of the foetus non-invasively by analysing foetal cells in maternal blood (Bianchi 1995).

Since late abortion is usually considered worse (more dangerous and also morally more questionable) than early abortion, early prenatal diagnosis is preferred. Modern medicine also offers a way in which to use prenatal diagnosis to 'avoid' termination. A case has been described in which in vitro fertilisation, gamete intrafallopian transfer and chorionic villus sampling were used for a couple who were carriers of beta-thalassaemia (Brambati *et al.* 1990). A quadruplet pregnancy resulted, and two of the foetuses were 'reduced' after chorionic villus sampling. The authors describe their method as a way to avoid termination, but I do not see anything but a technical difference between ordinary termination and 'reduction' in a multiple pregnancy.

Indications

Indications for prenatal diagnostic procedures can be divided into the following three classes: general, specific and ethnic risk factors.

General risk factors include advanced maternal age (being over 34 years of age at the time of delivery increases the risk for numerical chromosomal abnormalities) and demonstrated risks for certain abnormalities in a screening test (like elevated or reduced serum alpha-fetoprotein concentrations). Specific risk factors are identified in the family history, the history of previous pregnancies or the mother's medical history (D'Alton and DeCherney 1993). Ethnic risk factors refer to the fact that, in certain populations, the frequencies of some recessive genes are so high that screening for the carrier status directly or indirectly is considered justified. Today, the great majority of investigations are directed towards families in which the risk factor is general and thus first defined in statistical terms (Simola 1995).

Many prenatal diagnostic evaluations end up confirming that the foetus does *not* have the condition searched for (e.g. in the Nordic countries amniocentesis and chorionic villus biopsy lead to selective abortion in only 1.5–3.8% of cases (Brondum-Nielsen and Norgaard-Pedersen 1993).

Foetal sex determination without a history of sex-linked disease in the family may be the major indication for prenatal procedures in some parts of the world. For example, in India, ultrasonography or amniocentesis for that purpose is illegal, even though it is still common practice. The strong cultural pressure to have sons still exists and leads to abortions of female foetuses (Booth *et al.* 1994). A majority of geneticists in the USA also said in a survey in 1987 that they would perform prenatal diagnosis for sex selection. They justify their view by referring to women's autonomy, while their Indian colleagues mention social pressures to limit the population and the expected harm to unwanted girls (Boss 1993).

Consent for prenatal diagnosis

As with any medical examinations or research, consent is nowadays considered an essential prerequisite for prenatal investigations. The issue is not, however, as one-dimensional as sometimes presented.

Consent can be defined as 'the granting to someone the permission to do something he would not have the right to do without such permission' (Downie and Calman 1994, p. 245). In various contexts adjectives like 'informed', 'competent' or 'implied' are often associated with it.

Informed consent is the term used most often in health care, in both research and clinical settings. It is problematic, for example, in the sense that a layman's consent can hardly ever be 'fully' informed in the same way as that of the person responsible for the investigation or research. Also relevant is the question of side effects: how 'fully' are these to be described?

Competent consent refers to the ability of the patient or subject to understand the information given. The issue is two-sided in that it is not only a question of the mental capacity of the receiver of the information, but also very much an issue involving the quality of the information given.

Implied consent refers to the assumption that the person has given consent by coming to the doctor and asking for help or advice. Certainly people consent to *something* by making an appointment, but their views on *what* they consent to may differ from those of health care personnel.

Empirical research has pointed out some problems related to consent in prenatal examinations. Even though prenatal testing is experienced as voluntary, women report that it is difficult to decline such testing when it is offered (Sjögren and Uddenberg 1988), or it is experienced as a routine or self-evident act. A Finnish study showed, for example, that only one quarter of the women taking part in serum screening described actively deciding about their participation (Santalahti *et al.* 1998). In the same study 35 out of 91 women suggested, as an improvement, that screenees should receive more information, primarily about the conditions the screening can reveal and secondarily about the technical characteristics of the test. The authors noted also that, since public health nurses and hospital personnel were aware of the ongoing study, they may have paid special attention to the issues of consent and adequate information, and thus the results may have given a better picture than actually existed before the study. This is an example of how even the research process can influence practice. It also demonstrates the difficulties in obtaining a picture of what *really* happens in practice.

In a British study, routine consultations between midwives, obstetricians and pregnant women were tape-recorded and the way alpha-fetoprotein screening was presented was analysed (Marteau *et al.* 1992). The results showed that, in general, little information was provided about the test, the conditions screened for and the meaning of either a negative or positive test. It was also found that the screening was very often presented in such a way as to encourage women to undergo the test.

It has also been shown that the level of knowledge of the women who have been given information before being screened for Down syndrome is poor and concentrates on practical aspects of the test (Smith *et al.* 1994). For example, only one-third of the women had correct knowledge about such claims as 'Most women with positive results have normal babies' and 'Negative results do not guarantee that everything is all right with the baby' (both true).

Consent was not even sought in a study screening for haemoglobinopathies in pregnant women in Rochester, New York (Rowley *et al.* 1989). The authors justified their decision in the following way: 'Consent for screening was not routinely sought; providers agreed that obtaining truly informed refusal required counselling approaching that to be provided to identified carriers and many providers might have declined to participate if they had had to obtain it.' Altogether 18 907 pregnancies were screened during the study period and 810 (4.3%) were positive. Of these 551 (68%) came for counselling and the partner was tested in 315 (57%) cases. A prenatal diagnosis was offered to 53 persons and accepted by 25. Thus many of the testees never knew they had been tested, one-third of those who tested positive did not come for counselling, and in slightly more than half of the cases the partner was tested. Yet the authors concluded that 'these data indicate that women identified as hemoglobinopathy carriers during pregnancy accept and use genetic information' (Rowley *et al.* 1989, p. 157).

The reproductive autonomy model

The objectives of prenatal diagnosis and screening have been expressed in many ways, and it is possible to distinguish three different models or views on the primary objectives of these activities.

The first model can be called the patient welfare model due to its emphasis on maternal and foetal welfare. It has been argued that the 'primary purpose of prenatal diagnosis is the continuation of normal and wanted pregnancies in which the welfare of both mother and foetus is the prime consideration' (Campbell 1984, p. 1634). (What Campbell actually has in mind here, is, however, probably prenatal screening, not diagnosis.) While maternal and foetal welfare are good goals, they are not, however, necessarily the reason for prenatal screening. Another example of screening in health care reveals the problematic nature of the patient welfare model. According to the logic of the model, the purpose of, for example, mammographic screening would be the continuation and welfare of the lives of women who screen *negative*. However, the actual purpose of mammography screening is to discover and destroy early cancer.

By analogy, the purpose of prenatal screening would be to discover and destroy defective foetuses. Both cancer and the defective foetus are treated as something equally undesirable. And, further, if we accept Campbell's formulation, should we not engage in lots of screening activities to reassure people that they do *not* have this or that disease or condition? The theme of reassurance recurs later in the context of autonomy, but so far this formulation of the objective of prenatal diagnosis can be considered vague. At least the welfare of foetuses cannot be the primary purpose of prenatal screening since the foetuses for whom the whole system was established will probably lose their lives.

The second model has been named the public health model (Lippman 1994), and it sees prenatal screening and diagnosis as a means of reducing the frequency of selected birth defects and thus improving public health. The model has been powerful, and it is discussed in detail later in this chapter.

The third model is the reproductive autonomy model (Lippman 1994), which concentrates on the individual level and sees prenatal diagnosis mainly as a means to give women information to aid them in their reproductive choices.

The reproductive autonomy model can be considered a widely accepted standard in prenatal diagnosis and screening today, and several guidelines on both sides of the Atlantic have emphasised it. For example, American guidelines from 1979 for the ethical, social and legal issues of prenatal diagnosis aim at helping workers in this area to 'provide the most favorable circumstances for thoughtful, informed, morally responsible decision making by parents' (Powledge and Fletcher 1979, p. 169). The guidelines 'were developed in a moral framework favouring the protection of individual choice and the autonomy of parents' (Powledge and Fletcher 1979, p. 171). A recent American report states explicitly that 'in a society such as ours, autonomy far outweighs any public health considerations' (cited by Marteau 1995, p. 1216). The *Encyclopedia of Bioethics* emphasises that 'prenatal diagnosis is for the purpose of providing information to couples about what they can expect' (Evans *et al.* 1995, p. 989). In Great Britain the Royal College of Physicians has listed the following four objectives for prenatal diagnostic services (cited by Marteau 1995, p. 1216):

- to allow the widest possible range of informed choice to women and couples at risk of having children with an abnormality;
- to provide reassurance and reduce the level of anxiety associated with reproduction;
- to allow couples at risk to embark on having a family knowing that they may avoid the birth of seriously affected children through selective abortion;
- to ensure optimal treatment of affected infants through early diagnosis.

The general issue of autonomy is, of course, far too large to be dealt with in detail here, but a few things are worth mentioning. Firstly, the heavy emphasis on the principle of autonomy in modern bioethics is of American origin and has its roots in the Anglo-American law tradition that gives priority to individual over societal rights (Boss 1993). From a European, African or Asian perspective the picture of autonomy may look quite different.

While in Great Britain and northern Europe autonomy has been ranked almost as high as in the United States, southern European bioethics stresses different things. Patients in these countries are generally less concerned with their autonomy than with finding a doctor whom they can fully trust (Gracia 1993).

The systems of thought in many parts of the world favour collective rather than individual thinking, and this preference is reflected in decision-making. An example is a young rural woman in South Africa who, after childbirth, developed paralysis of the lower limbs and could not accept a lift to hospital because she had not consulted her mother (Qureshi 1997). In Japan, the family as a unit is preferred to the individual, and, for example, the diagnosis of cancer is revealed first to the family, which then decides whether the patient is told or not (S. Ohara, personal communication).

Secondly, emphasising parental autonomy in reproductive decisions may very strongly obscure other important issues. Concerning selective abortion, Boss (1993, p. 12) remarked that 'the discussion . . . has more often centered around who should decide, with the final decision generally resting with the mother, rather than the more basic question of whether the decision should be made at all and, if so, under what conditions or within what limitations'. Strong emphasis on autonomy may even lead to a more unstable policy concerning indications for prenatal diagnosis. Goodey (1997, p. 207) believes that ' "informed choice" is really a way of dumping on individual parents the moral responsibility for choices already made by the wider society, and perhaps the burden of challenging those choices'.

The reproductive autonomy model has been formulated in various ways with different emphases, and below I examine it in the form of the following claims: (1) prenatal diagnosis is a response to the request of pregnant women; (2) prenatal diagnosis provides reassurance of the health of the foetus to anxious parents; and (3) prenatal diagnosis enhances the control women have over their reproduction.

Response to a request

A central justification for the widespread offering of prenatal screening and diagnosis is that these methods are considered responses to the request of pregnant women. The exact opposite, however, has been suggested also (i.e. that the availability of prenatal screening and diagnosis has *created* the requests). There is, in fact, some empirical evidence to support the latter view. Press and Browner (1997) examined the spreading of the maternal serum alpha-fetoprotein (MSAFP) test in California and concluded that institutional and professional support for testing has yielded high rates of patient test acceptance. In California it is mandatory to offer MSAFP testing for every pregnant woman, and this practice has been interpreted to mean that it is standard care (Press and Browner 1997). The authors demonstrated also how the connection between abortion and MSAFP was absent when the test was described by the providers to the patients. Thus the 'very ethical issues of prenatal activity become obscured in the processes by which this screening test becomes accepted as routine' (Press and Browner 1997, p. 979).

A European study on the diffusion of four prenatal screening tests across Europe concluded more carefully that the 'demand for the test from individual consumers has always been said to be high, although the influence of the consumer is often difficult to document, and in the country reports must be derived from anecdotal comments' (Reid 1991, p. 41). According to the report, the diffusion of the tests is affected by the following three significant common factors: the importance of religion, the dependence on physicians' and consumers' knowledge and attitudes, and the degree of control exercised by governments over the development of the service.

The manner in which a test is offered to women may influence its uptake significantly. Only 10% uptake was reached when a carrier test for cystic fibrosis was offered in writing, but the uptake rose to 87% when the test was offered verbally with enthusiasm (Watson *et al.* 1991). In an article on informed consent and the screening for Duchenne muscular dystrophy (Parsons and Bradley 1994, p. 105) the authors speculated the following scenarios, where the offer for the test could be framed very differently:

- You want all the tests, don't you?
- You don't want the Duchenne test, do you?
- You do want the new Duchenne test, don't you?
- Have you thought about the new test? What have you decided to do?

Prenatal testing is usually offered by experts whose attitudes apparently have greatly affected the willingness of pregnant women's requests. In a study by Marteau *et al.* (1991) it was found that the willingness to have amniocentesis was associated with a less negative attitude towards the termination of an affected baby and a higher perceived risk of the foetus being abnormal, but *not* with actual age-related risks. There was no significant relation between the actual and perceived risk for abnormality.

The way the concept of risk is dealt with is interesting. The 35th birthday has become a turning point at which the pregnant woman becomes a risk case. At that age the risk for Down syndrome is 1/385, and for a chromosomal abnormality in general it is 1/202. Five years later it is 1/106 and 1/65, respectively (D'Alton and DeCherney 1993). Women who are 35 years old or older are considered as 'high risk' in this context. However, amniocentesis, which carries a risk between 1/100 and 1/200 for spontaneous abortion, is considered a 'safe' procedure (Kingston 1994). When professionals talk about risks in this way, it is not surprising that no significant relation exists between actual risk and perceived risk in the thinking of pregnant women.

Risk figures can also be experienced very differently. Firstly, even the formal way a risk figure is presented influences its interpretation. According to a study in which risk figures unrelated to genetic risk were presented to undergraduate psychology students, the percentages tended to be chosen as having greater magnitude than their equivalent proportions (Kessler and Levine 1987). In another study, respondents were asked to grade given risk percentages into the following four classes: high, moderate or low risk or cannot say (Somer *et al.* 1988). A risk of less than 1% was graded as high by 6% and low by 68% of the respondents. At the other extreme a risk of 50% was graded as high by 39%, moderate by 52% and low by 3% of the respondents. It is worth noting that there was no difference in risk perception with respect to the general education of the respondents.

Furthermore, the whole risk estimate, which is so central in the scientific part of the genetic counselling process, may have little meaning for the prospective mother or parents. For them there are only two outcomes: they will or will not have a defective child.

The issue of risk raises also the issue of paternalism: whose conception of the risk level is the 'right' one? Bosk (1992, p. 47) described a postclinic conference at a centre providing genetic counselling services and cited a medical doctor as follows: 'There are three different situations to worry about. Cases where parents accept a very high risk, cases where they deny there is any risk at all, and cases where they can't get the meaning of the risk clear in their own minds.' When is a risk 'very high', and when can it be said that the meaning of a risk is clear in one's mind?

A request for prenatal diagnosis and subsequent termination of pregnancy may be the result of external pressures on the woman or couple. If they feel that they can take care of the handicapped child but cannot trust society to do so after they are gone, the choice may be termination against their own wishes. According to Clarke (1990), the provision of prenatal diagnostic services for a particular condition may itself create a pressure to terminate an affected pregnancy: why else would there be such testing?

Commercial issues may also influence the uptake of prenatal diagnosis in countries where the private sector takes care of these activities. On a video presenting a prenatal diagnosis centre the narrator states:

you are pregnant, and like most pregnant women, you are wondering: 'will my baby be born healthy and normal?'. If your HEALTH care provider has told you that you are at INCREASED risk of having a child with a serious birth defect, prenatal diagnosis may offer you an answer to this question . . . Whether or not you decide to have a prenatal diagnosis, is up to you, but whatEVER your choice, try to keep in mind that most babies are born perfectly healthy. (Transcribed by Riitta Kärki from the documentary *The Cyborg Cometh*, A Big Table Film Company Production for Channel Four Television, presented on Finnish TV1 8 November 1995.)

This kind of rhetoric, which resembles that of commercial television, is further evidence to support the view that the availability of tests creates requests for prenatal screening and diagnosis and not necessarily vice versa.

The eagerness for prenatal diagnosis may also be viewed from the providers' side, as health professionals' willingness for technological solutions to all kinds of problems (Lippman 1994). Examples from other fields of medical technology show that once a new method (e.g. computer-assisted tomography) is available, new standards are produced concerning what ought to be available. This situation is probably true as well with prenatal diagnostic methods, the development of which creates new standards.

Angus Clarke, a geneticist, has expressed his worry about an obvious risk connected to prenatal diagnostic services. The feeling of parents when facing the fact that their foetus has a serious disorder is sadness, and this feeling is also, in part, shared by the person whose task is to break the bad news. However, at the same time, the geneticist may tend to have a sense of triumph at the diagnosis and subsequent termination. Clarke warns that the true justification of the procedure – the prevention of future suffering (of the disabled person or the family) when sought by the families concerned – may be obscured (Clarke 1990).

Reassurance

Although it is gross exaggeration to say that reassuring the great majority with normal results in prenatal testing would be the primary purpose of the activity, it is worth examining the role reassurance may have in the justification of prenatal diagnosis and screening.

Firstly, there is evidence that at least chromosomal and alpha-fetoprotein testing are reassuring to most women (Gates 1994).

Secondly, however, false positive results outnumber correct positive ones in most tests and cause anxiety, which is also well documented (Marteau 1995).

Thirdly, the reassurance of those receiving negative test results may be false, since, despite the information given before testing, there is a tendency among women tested to think that the test has ruled out more than it actually has.

Fourthly, women or parents often poorly understand the tests they undergo. Respondents in a Californian study on alpha-fetoprotein screening justified their accepting the test with comments like 'because I wanted to make sure my baby would be the healthiest that it could be' or 'I wanted to do anything that could help me or my baby' (Press and Browner 1994, p. 213). I assume that the comments did not refer to the possibility for advance preparations for neonatal surgery to repair meningomyelocele or hydrocephalus. A woman interviewed in a Finnish study commented in a similar way: 'I have the principle that all the tests which are done are done for my and my baby's best interests' (Santalahti *et al.* 1998). The test in question was serum screening for Down syndrome, and one may question what the woman meant by her 'baby's best interests'. I guess that she did not have an adequate picture about what she had taken part in but was sharing something that has been called 'collective fiction', in other words, situating the testing within the domain of routine prenatal care and denying its central connection to selective abortion and its eugenic implications (Press and Browner 1994).

Who controls prenatal diagnosis?

It is obvious that the introduction of prenatal diagnosis and screening has increased possibilities for controlling reproduction. It is, however, far less obvious where this control lies. The claim that it lies with pregnant women is only a half-truth.

The pregnant women – the people whom prenatal diagnosis mainly concerns – have not made the decisions about the conditions that are sought for. Individual pregnant women do not necessarily draw the line between 'normal, wanted' and 'abnormal, not wanted' in the same way as the medical community does. The latter is also far from uniform in its thinking. This has also been demonstrated empirically. In Canada, for example, female physicians were more liberal than their male colleagues with regard to access to amniocentesis and selective abortion. They also had a less directive relationship with their patients. The least and most directive specialities were obstetrics and paediatrics, respectively (Bouchard and Renaud 1997).

A grey area between foetuses with normal chromosomes and foetuses with serious defects leading to retardation or severe anomalies is the group with sex chromosome abnormalities. Most of them are compatible with normal life expectancy and actually often go undiagnosed. In a comparative study, which was performed in England and in Finland, it was found, for example, that a decision to terminate was made more often in Finland than in England and also more often when post-amniocentesis counselling was given by an obstetrician rather than a geneticist (Holmes-Siedle *et al.* 1987). The sample size in that study was small, but it shows how much cultural and religious factors and the counselling process itself influence women's decisions.

One form of control can also be seen in the way genetic disorders are described. Independently of each other, Lippman and Wilfond (1992) observed that, for cystic fibrosis and Down syndrome, the information provided to those considering genetic testing differs strikingly from that provided to those who have a child with one of these conditions. The overall information was correct in both circumstances, but the before-birth information was more negative than the after-birth information.

Parental control over reproduction may be seriously limited by economic constraints, especially in countries where health care is financed mostly through private insurance companies. In a case of a pregnant woman already with one child with cystic fibrosis the insurance company, a health maintenance organisation (HMO), agreed to cover prenatal testing but not the care of an affected child, who could have been aborted. The foetus was found to be affected and the HMO finally agreed to cover the child's treatment, but the initial policy of the HMO shows the limits of the control women themselves have over their pregnancies (Gates 1994). To my knowledge, so far there have been no cases in which insurance coverage has actually been rejected for a handicapped child whose diagnosis was known prenatally but who was not aborted. At least in the USA such a case would be highly political and create huge publicity.

The nature of the discourse determines the attitudes towards 'abnormal' foetuses. Children born with a disorder are considered 'failures' and the births as accidents where nature has failed to perform its natural selection, through which most abnormal foetuses abort spontaneously (Lippman 1994). The latter theme is common in the justification of selective abortion: it is considered the completion of the natural process (see Chapter 7).

In the beginning of the era of prenatal diagnosis there was serious disagreement about whether amniocentesis ought to be provided at all to couples who would not undergo abortion. Although the 'official policy' today states that, after prenatal diagnosis, there is total freedom of choice either to continue the pregnancy or to terminate it, practice again shows a different picture. Many doctors operate on the assumption that the only purpose of prenatal diagnosis is to detect foetuses with major anomalies so that they can be aborted (Hill 1986). Women can even be denied the right to diagnostic testing if they are not willing to abort in case of disability (Santalahti *et al.* 1996).

Prenatal diagnosis and screening are examples of new technologies that have raised vivid discourse in the feminist framework. Early feminist writings in the mid 1980s suggested that it was another 'male takeover' of female nature (Rapp 1994). No single simple feminist answer exists, however, for the question of the role of these new technologies in women's lives. They are potential tools both for liberation and for control over women's lives (Rapp 1994).

The public health model

Although the reproductive autonomy model has been said to dominate current thinking in genetics and medicine in general, contrasting views are still expressed more or less openly today. In the public health model either the general health and well-being of the population or economic factors are used as justification for prenatal diagnosis and screening. In the following discussion, I first examine arguments that have been presented to support the public health model. These are (1) the argument referring to public health, (2) the economic argument and (3) the 'medical view' argument.

Impact on public health

In the early days of prenatal diagnosis some very strict opinions were expressed in which not much room was left for individual autonomy. John Littlefield (1969, p. 722) wrote an editorial to the *New England Journal of Medicine*, in which he promoted the recently invented technique to perform prenatal chromosomal diagnosis: 'Perhaps it should be carried out routinely in older pregnant women exposed to an increasing risk of delivering a mongoloid infant.' Later he stated that 'society and the professions must appreciate and accept that the proper therapy now is for the family, and at times that means abortion' (Littlefield 1969, p. 723).

An eminent geneticist, Bentley Glass, who was the president of the American Association for the Advancement of Science, wrote in 1971 about future man: 'No parents will in that future time have a right to burden society with a malformed or a mentally incompetent child. Just as every child must have the right to full educational opportunity and a sound nutrition, so every child has the inalienable right to a sound heritage' (Glass 1971, p. 28).

A Swedish researcher Lars Svennerholm wrote one year later in a book about mental retardation: 'Nor is it any ethical problem to advise an abortion when a woman carries a male foetus with muscular dystrophy or haemophilia, but what about a female foetus who is a carrier of this defect? Up to this day, approximately 250 amniocenteses in connection with metabolic diseases have been performed. Already, a praxis has been formed: in the cases where there has been doubt whether the foetus is a carrier of or homozygous for the disease and there has been no time for a new test, a termination has been performed. Consequently, rather one abortion too many than the birth of a sick child.' (Translated and cited by Munthe (1996).)

These three quotations were from the early days of prenatal testing, but reference to public health as a justification of prenatal diagnosis has not disappeared. A report on population health outcomes by the Faculty of Public Health Medicine in the UK specifies as the objective of prenatal services to 'reduce the number of infants born with Down syndrome and neural tube defects' (cited by Marteau 1995, p. 1216).

The first three views represent overt paternalism, which is commonly rejected in current health care settings, at least in the USA, UK and northern Europe. The doctor's authority over matters other than strictly medical ones is no longer self-evident.

Paternalism has been defined as 'the power and authority one person or institution exercises over another to confer benefits or prevent harm for the latter regardless of the latter's informed consent' (Honderich 1995, p. 647). Paternalism can be divided into categories like soft and hard paternalism (Häyry 1991) or genuine, solicited and unsolicited paternalism (Wulff *et al.* 1986). An example of genuine or soft paternalism is a father who prevents his child from playing with matches. An example of solicited paternalism is a patient who explicitly gives the power of decision to the doctor. A morally problematic form of paternalism is hard or unsolicited paternalism in which the patient is not consulted when decisions concerning investigations or treatments are made.

It is, however, far too simple to regard paternalism as an on-off phenomenon. The encounter between the doctor and the patient is so complex that genuine *non-paternalism* may be unattainable. This complexity is obvious already in the preceding definition of paternalism. To be able to give fully informed consent would require substantial knowledge, which is usually unattainable in normal circumstances. The doctor or other health care professional is a gatekeeper who controls the amount of information given to patients, and this control as such contains an element of paternalism.

Glass's statement about future parents having no right to 'burden society with a malformed or a mentally incompetent child' represents, however, overt paternalism, which is hard to justify without much of the patient rights gained during past decades being thrown away. In the same way, Svennerholm has described an overtly paternalistic practice where doctors have made a *general* decision to abort in a 50-50 risk situation.

Another controversial issue in the preceding examples is the use of the word 'therapy' in the context of abortion. In fact, 'therapeutic abortion' is a commonly used term referring to the termination of pregnancy after prenatal diagnosis. I shall discuss the moral status of the foetus in later chapters, but a few remarks are relevant here.

It is more and more common to refer to the foetus as a patient or talk about foetal therapy. Whatever our view on foetal rights or foetuses as persons, it is agreed that foetuses can be treated on some occasions and that they are considered to have at least some rights. Littlefield referred to abortion as sometimes proper therapy for a family. This is a rather odd expression for eliminating something that, on another occasion, is considered a patient. Littlefield is right when he refers to the family as the target of the whole activity, but 'therapy' is not the proper term to describe it.

Economic argument

Another line of argument to support the public health model has been economic, although at the governmental level it has largely been considered unacceptable (Reid 1991). Numerous examples of direct reference to economic justification can, however, be found in the literature.

For example, Pauker and Pauker (1994, p. 1152) have discussed the question of what should be the age above which amniocentesis should be offered to all women. At the end of their article they wrote: 'Because limited resources now restrict the number of amniocenteses that can be performed and the number of couples who can be counselled, any restriction should reflect the risk in an individual pregnancy, not just the woman's age, and should be based on an analysis that includes economic costs of short- and long-term medical, social and home care for affected children, many of whom mature into physically and intellectually impaired adults.'

Chapple *et al.* wrote, in 1987, an article in which they concluded that the British Health Authorities should attach high priority to the setting up of DNA screening laboratories. They admitted that there would be enormous difficulties in conducting a cost–benefit analysis and that they did not consider the ethical issues at all. An implicit assumption behind the calculations seemed to be that those offered the services would fully participate and that in cases in which, for example, cystic fibrosis, beta-thalassaemia or haemophilia would be found, abortion would always follow.

The authors also wrote: 'As well as parental consent for termination of pregnancy, doctors involved in the care of affected families must consider the diseases sufficiently severe to warrant referral for termination' (Chapple *et al.* 1987, p. 1192). Talking about 'parental consent for termination' is particularly revealing. The idea of termination does not come from the pregnant woman or the couple but is *suggested* by the doctor. What level of severity justifies abortion is also a matter for the medical community to decide.

A third example comes from Finland, where policy decisions concerning health services are made locally by health committees, which consist mainly of laymen nominated on a political basis. In 1993 two gynaecologists and a medical geneticist proposed that serum screening be started in their area. The proposal listed factors to be considered when an appropriate screening programme is chosen. In the long run, savings were said to be expected because of the reduced number of intellectually disabled persons (Santalahti and Hemminki 1998).

Indirect reference to public health or economics is also common. For example, Dalgaard and Norby (1989, p. 324), when discussing autosomal dominant polycystic kidney disease (ADPKD) (which has nothing to do with intellectual disability), ended their article by stating: 'However, neither gene product manipulation nor gene therapy may become feasible for ADPKD in the foreseeable future. This stresses the importance of access to selective reproductive prevention as well as further development of conventional therapeutic measures.' In their review article on prenatal diagnosis D'Alton and DeCherney (1993, p. 118) wrote: 'Cost-effective screening is expected to be possible for many disorders, including cystic fibrosis.' The term 'cost-effective' has, in fact, been mentioned as one of the prerequisites for genetic screening (Simpson 1991). How it is measured is not obvious, and one may wonder whether it is implicitly assumed that defective foetuses are always or nearly always aborted and therefore the screening is cost-effective.

Anecdotal evidence also suggests that, in practice, doctors tend to think in terms of public health and the economy. After being told she carried a foetus with Down syndrome, a woman described her experience at an appointment with a doctor as follows:

My husband wanted to take rapid action to get rid of the problem and he had a good ally in the doctor. I became very angry. I was 41 years old, and I was told that, after the abortion I would certainly become pregnant again and that certainly the baby would be healthy. The doctor explained how expensive the tests are and how few defective foetuses are found. I understood that, if the foetus were aborted, my child would pay with its life because of the investigations done 'in vain' if it were healthy. Or if I would not agree to the abortion, I would be wasting society's money. (Puskala 1995; my translation from Finnish.)

The woman wrote her story when the child was 2 and a half years old, and it is, of course, impossible to form an objective picture of what happened at that appointment three years earlier. The actual conversation may have been less black-and-white than what she recalled, but her story describes the tendency of at least some members of the medical profession to think about prenatal screening as a population-level tool for prevention.

The preceding examples have one thing in common. The underlying assumption seems to be that, in all or nearly all cases, the diagnosis of the disease or handicap in question leads to abortion. In fact, the *very idea* of cost–benefit calculations includes this premise and can thus be considered to contradict the reproductive autonomy model. If the primary aim of prenatal diagnosis and screening were to enhance reproductive autonomy, the success of these activities would be measured in such terms, and the economic consequences would be *totally irrelevant.*

Another problem with most of the cost–benefit analyses is the omission of factors other than financial costs and benefits from the calculations. Some authors mention these and recognise also the ethical issues involved; others simply present monetary calculations.

An attempt has been made to combine the reproductive autonomy model with the cost–benefit analysis of a genetic screening programme (Modell and Kuliev 1991). In it a new model for the cost–benefit analysis of genetic services for thalassaemia is proposed. The model also takes into account non-financial costs and benefits.

The authors begin by listing some disadvantages of traditional cost–benefit analyses, which aim to show the superiority of prevention through the use of screening and prenatal diagnosis in financial terms only:

1 Patients and families are caused psychological harm by describing them as a financial burden to society.
2 Treatment and prevention should be seen as complementary aspects of a single policy, not as competing policies.
3 The traditional analyses seem to imply that prevention is better because it is cheaper. It should, however, be considered better only if people want it.
4 When costs are expressed in pounds per affected birth prevented, the implication is that the main objective in prenatal diagnosis is termination of affected pregnancies.

Thereafter, the authors describe their own suggestion in which the main benefit of a genetic screening programme is informed choice on the part of couples at risk. *Whatever* their choice, as long as they are informed and offered counselling, the aim has been achieved. The main cost of the service is termination of pregnancy. In the case of thalassaemia the financial cost of having a healthy child after selective termination of an affected foetus is 30% of the annual cost and 2% of the total (discounted) cost of treating a thalassaemic patient.

Modell and Kuliev admit that their attempt is only an outline that should be developed further. They have, however, shown that alternatives to the mainstream are possible.

'Medical view' argument

In another case history a clinical geneticist told a group of paediatricians and obstetricians about the difficulties of counselling in cases in which one relative has the fragile X syndrome, which leads to intellectual disability in 85% of male carriers but only 25% of female carriers. When describing the particular case of a healthy woman with the fragile X genotype, the geneticist stated: 'It would be hard to make her understand why, *according to the view of modern medicine*, a foetus with the same genotype as the mother, should be aborted . . . ' (my italics, I was present at the meeting).

The speaker did not explain what he meant by 'the view of modern medicine', but he seemed to think that there is a collective understanding of how situations like these should be handled. It is worth noting that his view came up spontaneously in a weekly meeting and thus probably represents the actual values that direct his work and thinking. If asked about his views in a separate interview, the picture might have been different.

In a British case a retired physician described a patient from the early 1960s who had severe asthma and became pregnant in spite of a sterilisation operation (Gregg 1994). The patient was a devout Roman Catholic and termination of pregnancy would have been out of the question. The case description goes on: 'While it might have been *medically correct* to advise termination of the pregnancy it would have been wholly inappropriate . . . ' (my italics). The doctor respected the autonomy of the patient, but at the same time his statement reveals his opinion that there is a common medical understanding about the conditions in which advice for termination should be given.

In another Finnish case an obstetrician described the patients of a postnatal ward in a weekly meeting (at which I was present). A 42-year-old woman had given birth to a child with Down syndrome and in relation to comments on this birth the statement: 'There are still those women who do not want to have amniocentesis' was made. The assumption of the speaker seems to be that, hopefully, as time passes, such women will no longer exist.

In all these examples the speakers seem to assume a collective understanding about issues that are more of a moral than a scientific nature. Is there such collective understanding and what could be its nature?

It may be useful to separate the realms of facts and values when this question is dealt with, although it is obvious that, in medicine if anywhere, these realms are inseparable.

The view the medical community often wants to give of itself is that of a unanimous and unified collective of scientifically oriented individuals. Medical science is seen as the true basis of the practice of medicine, and the new paradigm of evidence-based medicine is considered a means of truly scientific practice. This may be the impression if one looks only at textbooks and major journals, especially in the English language. But looking a little further, particularly at medical practice in various parts of countries dominated by Western medicine, gives a totally different picture (Payer 1990). The variance of practices and even the spectrum of diagnoses are huge, and the picture of a unanimous collective collapses.

No doubt, there is also something that might be called common understanding with respect to many moral issues in medicine. This understanding is exemplified by various codes accepted, for example, by the World Medical Association. However, in a multitude of moral issues, the medical community is far from unanimous, and there is great variability between countries, cultures and specialities.

What is particularly interesting in the two examples that were just presented is that the speakers assume something, and that something *directly contradicts* the view expressed explicitly in several guidelines and codes. This situation raises the question of whether there is, in addition to the official view expressed in textbooks and guidelines, a hidden common morality that is expressed in daily practice.

It has been said that there are three ways of describing what a physician does. If he or she is asked how a problem should be handled, the answer may refer to textbooks or what the doctor thinks should be done. The third description is what he or she actually does in such situations. The same may be true in moral issues, the third way representing the hidden common morality that finds its expression in the actual daily practice of physicians.

Additional critical views

In addition to the preceding arguments concerning various aspects of the reproductive autonomy and public health models, there are some issues worth mentioning that do not refer specifically to any of the models. These issues are the slippery slope argument, the relationship between prenatal diagnosis and eugenics, and the impact of prenatal diagnosis on the lives of the disabled.

Slippery slope

The slippery slope argument means that, although a practice may be unobjectionable in one type of case, if it is once permitted, its use will inevitably be extended to other, more morally dubious cases (Honderich 1995). The inevitability supposed is not logical by nature but is, instead, based on a certain view of human nature that assumes people always want more than they have (Honderich 1995).

The slippery slope argument has been used commonly in medical ethics, especially in discussions concerning euthanasia and abortion. The problem with the argument is that it describes something that has happened in a certain historical setting, but it cannot forecast that, in a future setting, a similar slippery slope will logically be the outcome.

The most popular example of an actual slippery slope is the Nazi euthanasia programme which had its roots in the psychiatric reform and poor economics of the 1920s (Burleigh 1994). Starting with compulsory sterilisation in the interest of racial fitness it gradually grew into a systematic murder programme for 200 000 mentally ill or physically disabled people and, later, 6 million Jews in the 'Final Solution'.

Other examples of slippery slopes that are offered in medical ethics are the practice of euthanasia in The Netherlands and the practice of abortion in the countries that liberalised their abortion laws in the 1960s and 1970s. Both of these examples fail, however, to prove that an actual extension of a limited practice has taken place. While it is true that a small number of euthanasia cases occur in The Netherlands without explicit consent of the patient, it is not known what the situation was before. Thus nothing can be said about the possible *change* in the situation. A standard argument against abortion maintains that a substantial increase in the number of abortions has taken place in the countries in which more liberal abortion laws have been introduced (Sutton 1990). This argument fails also, since, in fact, empirical data can be provided that show a *decrease* in the number of abortions. For example, in Finland the yearly number of abortions has decreased from 20 000 in the early 1970s to 10 000 in the 1990s.

What form would the slippery slope argument take in the context of prenatal diagnosis and how powerful would it be? The formulation of the argument could be as follows: if prenatal diagnosis and selective abortion are applied in the first phase to severely handicapping conditions, they will inevitably be applied to milder and milder handicaps and eventually to qualitative characteristics that, by no serious definition, can be considered handicaps.

In the time scale of the 30 years during which prenatal diagnosis has been available, no slippery slope has been recognised, at least in general policies concerning the severity of the conditions justifying prenatal diagnosis. Down syndrome was one of the first conditions diagnosed, and in all these years a discussion about whether it is a serious handicap or not has been going on. Foetal sex determination without a history of sex-linked disease in the family has not become a widely accepted practice in Western countries, and the practice in India can hardly be considered to support the slippery slope argument. Thus the argument has turned out not to support a critical view of prenatal diagnosis and screening.

Prenatal diagnosis and eugenics

The connection between prenatal diagnosis and screening on one hand and eugenics on the other hand is sometimes discussed and mostly denied by geneticists. The word 'eugenics' has bad connotations that lead thoughts to the Nazi era, and thus the eagerness to dissociate from it is understandable. On the other hand, in 1991, an editorialist of *Nature* wrote: 'The eugenic issue, to which the present practice of amniocentesis followed (sometimes) by abortion is a crude approach, is similarly unstoppable in the long run' (*Nature* 1991, p. 591). I have already briefly discussed the historical development of the attitudes towards intellectual disability (see Chapter 4 on prevention) and shall return to the concept of eugenics for a while.

Eugenics can be defined either as 'a science concerned with the control of hereditary traits through selective human mating' or as 'the deliberate control, by law or social pressure, of the perpetuation of human genetic traits' (*The New Grolier Multimedia Encyclopedia* on CD-ROM, Release 6, 1994).

Positive eugenics aims at increasing the reproduction of individuals considered the most valuable to society. A modern version of this kind of thinking is the founding of sperm banks, which select their donors with strict IQ criteria. Another example of present-day positive eugenics is found in Singapore, where it was decided in 1983 to offer educational advantages to children born to educated women (*The New Grolier Multimedia Encyclopedia* 1994).

Negative eugenics aims at decreasing the reproduction of individuals who are considered genetically handicapped. The commonest means of negative eugenics has been compulsory sterilisation, a common practice in many countries until the 1960s. A form of present-day negative eugenics is China's 1995 Law on Maternal and Infant Health Care (Jones 1996, *Nature Genetics* 1997). Under Article 10 of the law, people diagnosed with a 'genetic disease of a serious nature' are asked to take (unspecified) long-term contraceptive measures or to be sterilised. Article 16 of the same law is less specific but implies compulsory prenatal testing and pressure on women to abort under certain circumstances.

These examples of positive and negative eugenics are rather extreme, but it is worth looking at the preceding definitions of eugenics in light of the aims of genetic counselling and prenatal diagnosis today. Some current programmes to prevent serious genetic disease fit the definition of eugenics as a 'science concerned with the control of hereditary traits through selective human mating'. Examples of these programmes are screening for the Tay–Sachs gene among Ashkenazi Jews and the thalassaemia gene among Cypriots (D'Alton and DeCherney 1993). Both programmes have been successful in decreasing the incidence of these diseases.

If eugenics is 'deliberate control, by law or social pressure, of the perpetuation of human genetic traits', the public health genetics of today can be seen to share its aim. Today, control by law is mostly out of the question, but social pressure has been demonstrated in several studies in many countries. It can also be said that the agency of eugenic control has shifted from society to the individual (Boss 1990).

What is the effect of current practice in prenatal diagnosis on the human gene pool in general? Abortion of affected foetuses with *chromosomal* disorders will not affect significantly the gene pool since the disorders are not usually inherited but are results of errors in gametogenesis. Abortion of foetuses with *multifactorial* or *polygenic* disorders has also little or no known effect on the gene pool since other factors besides genes have an obvious influence on the status of the individual.

Prenatal diagnosis and selective abortion will probably reduce the frequency of *dominant monogenic* disorders like Huntington's disease. However, not all families are willing to take this path, and fresh mutations are also occurring that cannot be anticipated.

A greater part of severe monogenic disorders are inherited as a *recessive* trait. If it is true that the availability of prenatal diagnosis increases the number of healthy children who replace the foetuses lost through selective abortion, then the number of abnormal genes in the human gene pool actually *increases*, since the healthy children are carriers of the recessive genes (Boss 1990).

The application of prenatal diagnosis and selective abortion is thus *dysgenic*, not *eugenic*, when the total effect on the human gene pool is considered. The magnitude of this dysgenic effect is, however, so small that it would take over 200 years for it to make any measurable impact (Jackson 1990). Whether we want to utilise prenatal diagnosis or not has to be judged on other grounds.

Impact on the disabled

The standard argument from the disability activists against prenatal screening is that it is 'selective genocide against the disabled' (i.e., it has a serious negative effect on the lives of the disabled, who either are among us already or who are born in the era when prenatal diagnosis is possible; this is a term used by the disability movement itself; it appears in a citation from Luker (*Abortion and the Politics of Motherhood*) in Bosk 1992, p. 25). On the other hand, proponents of prenatal screening have argued that its widespread availability will have little or even a positive effect on the lives of the disabled. The latter view has been justified by references to the increased awareness of carrier statuses for various diseases, which might blur the distinction between the affected and the unaffected. This view has been presented by Bernadette Modell, who has been cited by Marteau and Drake (1995). In the following discussion I first consider possible discrimination as a practical issue and then analyse the philosophical argument at the conceptual level.

Little empirical research has been done so far and not much can be said about the actual effect of prenatal screening and diagnosis on public opinion. Marteau and Drake (1995) studied the influence of genetic screening on the attributions that are given for disability. According to the attribution theory more help is given when dependency is attributed to factors such as lack of ability on the victim's part than when it is attributed to a lack of effort on the victim's part. In the study pregnant women, geneticists, obstetricians and a general sample of men and women in three countries (the UK, Germany and Portugal) responded to two case vignettes in which a woman gave birth to a child with Down syndrome. In the first case the woman declined the offer for testing; in the second no test was offered by the hospital. In all the groups of respondents the woman who declined the test was attributed more blame for the disability of her child than the other woman was. An interesting finding was that the geneticists were the least likely to attribute blame following the birth of a child with Down syndrome. The authors widely discussed the limitations and implications of the study and noted that, while genetic screening may influence attributions for the birth of a child with a disability, it is not known how these attributions differ from those made before screening was widely available.

In a French follow-up study of a cohort of Down syndrome foetuses and newborns, a larger-than-expected number of unexplained deaths was observed (Julian-Reynier *et al.* 1995). Due to the lack of detailed data about the deaths, the authors were cautious about their conclusions, but they discussed the possibility that parents and professionals may feel more justified than in the past for not providing Down syndrome children with the necessary care.

I mentioned earlier the finding of Lippman and Wilfond (1992) about the differences between the information given about Down syndrome in the screening context and that given to parents who have given birth to a child with Down syndrome. One can only imagine the feelings of the parents in a situation in which the screening test has been negative and still a child with Down syndrome has been born. However, the life of the child need not be miserable, as was demonstrated in a documentary film describing such a family (shown on Finnish TV, Channel 1 on 17 March 1999; my translation). Santeri, a boy with Down syndrome, was born after negative serum, nuchal translucency and ultrasound screening tests. When he was a few months old, his parents were interviewed. Santeri's father described the initial shock the parents experienced when their son was born, but added:

Afterwards it feels rather strange that Down syndrome is so widely screened for . . . It is, of course, the most common chromosomal aberration . . . Somehow we had a picture in our minds that it must be the most serious or terrible thing because it is so much screened for. Actually it was a surprise for us how normal life can be, at least with a small boy with Down syndrome.

Santeri's mother gave her own interpretation of what had happened:

Santeri decided to cheat us in these tests and show that there's enough room in the world for a guy like him. 'I don't want to go away', was his message.

This case history is a beautiful example of an individual whose life will probably be happy although his parents were originally determined not to have an intellectually disabled child if the screening tests had revealed such.

Empirical research or case studies do not, of course, settle the issue of possible discrimination against the disabled. It is possible, however, to picture some negative outcomes on the lives of the disabled. The following potential causes of increased discrimination have been presented: (1) a decrease in the numbers of disabled people and (2) a change for the worse in social attitudes towards the disabled (Gillam 1999).

The number of disabled people will not, however, decrease significantly in the foreseeable future. Disability in general is, to a great extent, due to factors other than genetic or prenatal circumstances, and current prenatal screening methods detect only a few causes of disability. In addition, the trend to have children at an older age may dilute the effect of screening on the birth prevalence of, for example, Down syndrome.

Moreover, the mere reduction in the number of disabled people cannot directly cause increased discrimination since such a causal link would mean that an *increase* in the number would necessarily bring about *less* discrimination.

In general, the extent of discrimination against disabled people has decreased significantly over the past 20 to 30 years (Gillam 1999). A negative change in the attitudes due to prenatal screening is, however, possible. The birth of a child with a disability will increasingly become a matter of conscious choice, and in this environment parents who take that choice may be seen as acting irresponsibly. This situation may lead to some people being considered accidents that should never have happened. The attitudes of part of the medical community (see the preceding section 'Medical view' argument) show that the fears of some disability activists should be taken seriously. But even so the change is not always inevitable. There is no *necessary* connection between discriminatory outcomes and prenatal screening. It is plausible to think of disability as an accident without thinking of a disabled person as an accident.

I have so far dealt with the empirical or practical aspects of the discrimination argument. An analysis at the conceptual level has recently been presented by John

Harris, who argues against a necessary connection between prenatal screening and the quality of life of the disabled (Harris 1998*b*). In many questions related to the ethics of prenatal diagnosis, I disagree with him (see Chapter 7), but in this question I find his main idea plausible.

Harris points out that we should not confuse two questions: (1) is it wrong to prefer a non-disabled person to a disabled one and (2) is it wrong to prefer to produce a non-disabled individual rather than a disabled one? With Harris, I answer without further argument 'yes' to the first question, although there are, of course, examples in real life where non-disabled persons are preferred to disabled ones.

The second question is more problematic, and Harris modifies it by dividing it into seven sub-questions: Is it wrong to prefer to produce a non-disabled child and attempt to achieve that preference:

(a) by wish fulfilment
(b) by behaviour modification
(c) by postponement of conception
(d) by therapy (including gene therapy)
(e) by selecting between preimplantation embryos
(f) by abortion
(g) by infanticide.

It is probable that there would be wide agreement in the answers to questions (a) through (e). There is obviously nothing wrong in wishing to have a non-disabled child (a). The modification of maternal behaviour (b), for example, the use of alcohol during pregnancy, or the postponement of conception (c), for instance, in the case of on-going cancer therapy, are also easily acceptable means of avoiding disability. Again, if there is a safe form of therapy (d), like the diet in PKU, there should be no moral problems in trying to avoid disability. The same holds true for preimplantation techniques (e), if they are safe and accepted in general.

The really controversial questions are (f) and (g). I shall deal with the general moral issues of abortion and infanticide more in Chapter 8 and concentrate here on abortion as a *method* to avoid disability.

If abortion on demand is accepted, the moral status of the foetus is somehow considered lower that that of an infant or child, even in the case of *any* foetus, with or without a condition leading to disability. If, on the other hand, abortion is prohibited because the foetus is granted the same moral status as an infant or child, this prohibition is not dependent on the disability status of the foetus.

Screening for PKU is considered unproblematic because there is a relatively easy way to prevent intellectual disability from developing in these children. If there were a similarly easy way to prevent disability in children with Down syndrome, there would hardly be any parents who would say no to such therapy. The problem is that there is no such therapy.

The point here is that there is no *necessary* connection between the means of trying to avoid disability and the way living disabled people are treated or respected in a society. The disagreements over the legitimacy of aborting disabled foetuses are disagreements over the legitimacy of abortion, not disagreements about attitudes towards disability or disabled people (Harris 1998*b*).

There are thus no empirical or conceptual reasons for a necessary connection between screening for disability and the lives of the disabled. The fears of disabled people are not, however, unjustified. The signals society gives in the context of screening (e.g. in emphasising economic savings as a justification for screening) may have a negative impact on the lives of the disabled. In addition, some hidden attitudes of the medical community may have a similar effect, and the possibility should not be ignored. Morally acceptable use of prenatal screening and diagnosis precludes that these possible negative effects be acknowledged and countered as far as possible (Gillam 1999).

Concluding remarks

Intellectual disability is the common denominator in a great majority of cases in which prenatal diagnosis and screening take place today. I have pointed out several problems with these practices and their justifications and shall summarise them briefly here.

Informed consent for prenatal diagnosis is difficult to obtain in practice; at least so far there are serious shortcomings. Medical and other health care personnel do not share a uniform view on this issue either, and the tests have often turned into a routine, which may be difficult to resist.

Prenatal screening and diagnosis are sometimes responses to the requests of pregnant women. The influence of consumers on the development of these technologies is, however, difficult to document, and it has been suggested that the availability of prenatal screening and diagnosis creates these requests. Important modifiers of practice are also experts' attitudes and the way tests are offered. The concept of risk is a central issue, but it is often poorly understood and can also be used in a manipulative manner to influence the uptake of tests.

There is evidence of both correct and false reassurance being given to women by prenatal testing. Evidence also indicates that there are psychological problems related to false positive results and that women poorly understand the tests they undergo.

Prenatal diagnosis has created a possibility to control reproduction in a powerful way that is unique in history. The control, however, is not necessarily with the pregnant women. The medical community decides what conditions are severe enough to be sought for and considered for termination. How this activity is financed varies from country to country, and evidence shows a willingness on the part of insurance companies to take control.

Justifying prenatal diagnosis and screening by referring directly to public health has not been popular during the past two decades, and earlier overtly paternalistic views on the regulation of reproduction have disappeared. Direct or indirect references to public health, and especially economics, are, however, common. There seems also to be a hidden collective view shared by many physicians about the 'right' behaviour of women in the context of prenatal diagnosis. This view has also been expressed repeatedly by one of the inventors of DNA, James Watson, who in 1993 opined that: '... [genetic testing] would make possible the routine diagnosis of vast numbers of genetic conditions, which should be eliminated by abortion ... it is a true act of moral cowardice to allow children to be born with known genetic defects' (Lucassen 1998, p. 1004). In a more recent contribution to *Time* magazine, Watson wrote 'There is, of course, nothing pleasant about terminating the existence of a genetically disabled foetus. But doing so is incomparably more compassionate than allowing an infant to come into the world tragically impaired' (Watson 1997, p. 86). The author did not specify the terms 'genetically disabled' and 'tragically impaired', but a message like this from a great authority in the field reveals something of a common hidden attitude.

There is no necessary connection between the practices of prenatal screening and the quality of life of the disabled who are either already among us or who are born in the era when prenatal diagnosis is possible. On the other hand, the attitudes of society and the medical community may negatively influence the lives of these people, and the fears expressed by the disability movement should be taken seriously.

The new inventions in prenatal diagnosis and screening have no doubt helped a multitude of families with their extremely difficult reproductive decisions. At the same time they have created a new set of moral problems that must be faced by the medical and scientific community, the families and society as a whole. One crucial setting in which these problems are faced is genetic counselling, and it will be my next topic.

6

Genetic counselling

Genetic counselling is 'what happens when an individual, a couple or a family asks questions of a health professional [the genetic counsellor] about a medical condition or disease that is, or may be, genetic in origin' (Clarke 1994, p. 1). The focus may be back in time (e.g. when a family is seeking an explanation for what has happened in the past) or forward in time (e.g. when a couple wants to know about their reproductive options). The 'patients' or clients are generally healthy, and with a few exceptions the whole clinical genetic practice is not involved with therapy. As Angus Clarke expressed it: 'We dispense words, not tablets' (Clarke 1997a, p. 165). Clarke is a clinical geneticist himself and thus an 'insider'. The American sociologist Charles L. Bosk has given an 'outsider's' view, which summarises some of the tensions of the process: 'Genetic counselling as a service is generally a matter of transferring information to individuals who request it, and then leaving those individuals alone to make the tragic choices based on that information' (Bosk 1992, p. xix).

Counselling centres were started in the USA as part of the eugenics movement already in 1915. This was not, however, counselling in the above sense; instead it coincided with the prevailing eugenic ideology. In the 1930s interest in genetic counselling declined because of the greater emphasis on the role of the environment in human behaviour (Hoedemaekers 1998). Later, after World War II, genetic counselling in the above sense was developed partly as a reaction against eugenics (Chadwick and Ngwena 1992).

The process of genetic counselling can be divided into five phases (Clarke 1994). Firstly, the counsellor listens to the clients and tries to determine what their questions are. Secondly, the diagnosis of the affected individual is confirmed or clarified as far as possible. Sometimes the definitive diagnosis is not found, and the only conclusion may be that the condition appears to be inherited as a recessive trait and thus the probability of recurrence in future pregnancies is 25%.

Thirdly, existing information is communicated to the clients. If possible, the background and education of the clients are taken into account. The third phase may end the process, but often the clients also wish to discuss the implications of the information they have received. The discussion is the fourth phase, and the focus can be, for example, on the consequences of either continuing a pregnancy or terminating it. It may also concern the therapeutic options available for the condition in question.

The fourth phase often ends the counselling process, but sometimes a fifth phase follows in which postcounselling is given by the counsellor. It may be supportive by nature, or sometimes it may even involve active participation in the care of patients, if the counsellor is at the same time a specialist in that area.

The background of the counsellors is often in medical genetics, but, to a greater degree, particularly in the USA, a specific profession of genetic counsellors has developed. People coming into the field may have a background in, for example, nursing or social work. Only a few clinical geneticists with a medical background have formal training in psychotherapy or counselling in a broad sense (Clarke 1997a). The content of the counselling process certainly depends on the background of the counsellor, but Bosk (1992) may have been right in stating that the emphasis in genetic counselling is quite clearly on genetics as a science, rather than on counselling as a relational process.

Goals

The goals of clinical genetics in general are far more numerous than those of genetic counselling in particular. The difference has not been obvious to the activists of the disability movement, who argue that the whole discipline has been established to avoid the existence of people like themselves.

In addition to the provision of information about the present pregnancy and future reproductive risks and options, the following activities are covered in the field of clinical genetics (modified from Clarke 1993):

1 To cooperate with other specialists in setting an early and precise diagnosis of the condition in question.
2 To cooperate with other specialists in the screening for complications of a genetic disease.
3 To provide social and practical support for individuals and families with a genetic disease.
4 To take part in research aiming at new specific therapies for genetic diseases.

In his article about the role of genetic counselling, Clarke (1993, p. 47) also mentioned the following:

5 'The reduction of "handicap", itself a social construct, by working to minimise the stigma associated with disability and handicap, hoping to develop the self-esteem of affected individuals.'

While the clinical genetics community probably agrees with points 1 to 4, point 5 is more controversial, and at least at the practical level it is not experienced as a central activity among geneticists.

The goals of genetic counselling are narrower and they concentrate for the most part on the future reproductive options of the clients. The following two key roles are identified in all the definitions: the communication of factual information and aid given to couples to help their decision-making (Marteau *et al.* 1994*b*).

The contradiction between the public health model and reproductive autonomy model, which were discussed in the previous chapter, is obvious also here. Although many geneticists would like to divorce themselves from the former, it may not be possible. There is, namely, a *logical* connection between genetic counselling as part of medical genetics and the incidence of genetic disease (Chadwick 1993). The fact that a screening programme has been established shows that it is considered good by both society and the medical community and that it is considered undesirable to have a genetic disease.

Giving a role to public health genetics does not imply, however, that any means can be used to achieve better genetic health among a population. Here there is a role for reproductive autonomy, which can be seen as a condition that determines the way objectives of public health genetics are pursued (Chadwick 1993).

When is genetic counselling successful?

The success of a medical activity can be measured in many ways. The outcome may be lives saved, life-years gained, quality-adjusted life-years gained, money saved or satisfaction of the patients gained. Genetic counselling is unique in the sense that none of these methods fits well as a measure of its success.

The number of selective abortions after prenatal diagnosis would be a simple numeric outcome, which could, although with methodological difficulties, be translated into financial savings attained. Choosing this measure would represent the public health model of prenatal diagnosis in its purest form. As we have seen, however, as the only justification for prenatal diagnosis and screening, the public health model seriously overlooks the autonomy of the clients or patients involved. The empirical evidence referred to suggests that, even without such a numeric outcome as an explicit measure, some clinicians think in terms of the public health model and also transfer their thinking to their clients.

If the public health model does not provide a measure of the success of genetic counselling, what are the alternatives? The lives gained through the possibility for prenatal diagnosis, the general workload of the units giving counselling, or client satisfaction are possible outcomes (Clarke 1990).

It may be true that, in many cases, couples would reject the idea of having more children *without* prenatal diagnosis, and thus, as a result of this activity, there is a 'gain' of healthy children. Their number is, however, beyond any quantification, and, even if it were possible to estimate it, the task would be to compare the number of lives thus gained with the potential number of lives with disability that are avoided. It is hard to imagine what the unit of measurement would be in such comparisons. What is more important, however, is that monitoring the success of genetic counselling this way would entail imposing *a value judgement upon particular reproductive behaviours* (Clarke 1997a). This, again, would be an expression of a public health model, which would not respect the autonomy of individual clients.

Could the workload of a genetic counselling service serve as a criterion for success? Certainly it would describe the activity but not in terms of the goals, had they been explicitly set or not.

Client satisfaction could easily be measured by, for example, questionnaires, but as a measure of the success of genetic counselling this procedure is highly questionable. For example, should only the actual clients be asked about genetic counselling or should the general public be regarded as potential clients? And if the clients would show satisfaction, it would be restricted to the activity whose content has been determined by the medical community, not by the general public. What about the dissatisfaction associated with the lack of available information or with unwelcome information (Clarke 1997a)? Part of these problems could be solved by adopting the 'retrospective assessment of satisfaction' approach suggested by Clarke (1997a). Genetic counselling would be evaluated with the following three questions:

1 Were you satisfied with the service provided at the time? Was the service efficient and convenient to use?
2 What changes have occurred in your expectations of the genetic counselling service since your referral?
3 With hindsight, how satisfied are you with your experience of the genetic counselling service? If you went through a diagnostic process, was this of any use or value, even if no diagnostic certainty was achieved? Did the service meet the expectations that you now think you 'should' have had at the time of your referral?

This rather complicated approach has the advantage of acknowledging the possible mismatch between the client's initial expectations and the actual possibilities the service can provide. While this approach may succeed in measuring a certain aspect of the outcome of genetic counselling quite well, a global outcome measure for the entire process of genetic counselling may be unattainable (Clarke 1997a), and, no matter how the goals of genetic counselling are expressed, its impact on reproductive outcome is small. Precounselling reproductive intentions, rather than counselling, determine the outcome in families seeking counselling (Kessler and Levine 1989).

Directive or non-directive counselling?

The principle of non-directiveness was presented in the early days of genetic counselling. The term was borrowed from the general approach to counselling in the client-centred therapy developed by Carl Rogers in the 1940s (Clarke 1997*b*). Although non-directiveness was accepted generally as a principle, the practice of genetic counselling was something else (Michie *et al.* 1997*a*). For example, one of the pioneers in British clinical genetics, C. O. Carter, adopted the practice of encouraging parents with low or moderate risks (less than 1 in 20) by saying that 'in your place I would be prepared to take the risk' (Carter *et al.* 1971). The discussion section in a paper, also from the early 1970s, describing a consumer's view on genetic counselling opens by stating: 'Genetic counselling is preventive medicine and should be so regarded' (Leonard *et al.* 1972, p. 437). The paper was written by professionals in the field, not by representatives of consumers.

Follow-up studies done in the 1960s and 1970s indicate that counselling at that time was quite directive. The outcome of genetic counselling was measured in terms of, for example, whether the clients had accepted the counsellor's conclusions or whether the reproductive outcome was the one suggested by the counsellor (Michie *et al.* 1997*a*).

During the past 15 years non-directive genetic counselling has more unanimously been considered as an aim. For example, the *Code of Ethics* of the National Society of Genetic Counsellors (in the USA, cited by White 1998) states the following:

The counsellor–client relationship is based on values of care and respect for the client's autonomy, individuality, welfare and freedom. The primary concern of genetic counsellors is the interests of their clients. Therefore, genetic counsellors strive to:

Respect their client's beliefs, cultural traditions, inclinations, circumstances, and feeling.

Enable their clients to make informed independent decisions, free of coercion, by providing or illuminating the necessary facts and clarifying the alternatives and anticipated consequences.

Non-directiveness is an aim on this side of the Atlantic as well, although it has been admitted that, in connection with prenatal diagnosis, it may be unattainable (Clarke 1991). In a cross-cultural study among 1053 medical geneticists in 18 nations, a great majority (92–94%) regarded non-directive approaches to counselling as appropriate (Wertz and Fletcher 1988). More directive approaches were preferred in two East European countries (Hungary and the German Democratic Republic), but the study was done in the 1980s and later political changes have possibly decreased the differences.

Before turning to the contents of the concepts 'directive' and 'non-directive', I should first mention three issues. Firstly, the situations in which genetic counselling take place are very different, depending on the initiator of the process. If the client has contacted a genetic service for advice, the setting resembles a standard clinical encounter between a physician and a patient, and the issue is very much the same as with paternalism. By asking for advice, the client expresses a wish and may implicitly or explicitly give up a part of his or her autonomy. If, however, the initiator of the process is society in the form of a screening test, then a certain amount of 'structural' directiveness is introduced. Merely making prenatal screening and diagnosis available may send the message that they should be used (Clarke 1997*b*). Then it is not only the values of the counsellor that should be considered, but also the values of society and professional bodies that have made the screening possible. The *environment* may be directive, and a more directive mode of counselling may be needed to counteract the directiveness of the environment (Hoedemaekers 1998).

Secondly, a few words should be said about the reasons why non-directiveness has become such a standard or cornerstone of genetic counselling. The first reason is obvious. It is the strong position autonomy has in current health care ethics. Secondly, as mentioned in the beginning of this chapter, genetic counselling developed partly as a reaction to the abuses of human genetics in Europe and North America during the first half of this century (Clarke 1997*b*). Thirdly, an emotional explanation may be that non-directiveness may help the clients keep an emotional distance from the decisions they make (Clarke 1997*a*) and also help them maintain distance from the politics of second trimester abortion (Bosk 1992). Fourthly, it has also been suggested that the principle of non-directiveness can be viewed as an attempt to avoid the difficulty of defining a general goal or objective of genetic counselling (Michie *et al.* 1997*a*).

Thirdly, the very idea of non-directive counselling contains an internal contradiction. In Bosk's words: 'A commitment to non-direction requires a certain reticence to explore issues that patients keep closed. Yet a commitment to decisions that "patients are comfortable with" requires a certain amount of unpleasant prying if only to assure that the comfort presented is genuine' (Bosk 1992, p. 123).

What, then, do we actually mean when we talk about directiveness and non-directiveness? It is worth noting that a definition of either of these terms has been missing from the discussions about the nature of genetic counselling. The underlying assumption seems to be that the terms are understood in a uniform and non-problematic way.

In a recent empirical study on directiveness in genetic counselling an operative definition of directiveness was provided: 'Directions or advice that the counsellor suggests to the client in regard to specific behaviours or making decisions. Directions or advice about the client's views, attitudes or emotions' (Michie *et al.* 1997*a*). The statements of the counsellors were further classified into the categories advice, evaluation and enforcement. Examples are statements like 'It'd be sensible if you spoke to Michael and Carol about this' or 'We would recommend that you had the ultrasound screening' for advice, 'That is what we would consider quite a high risk' for evaluation and 'I think you've made the right decision' for reinforcement.

Some methodological issues are problematic in this study, but the results show that all consultations contained at least two directive statements. There were large individual differences in rated directiveness, and, interestingly, there were more evaluative statements in the consultations conducted by counsellors who had received counselling training than in the consultations by those who had not received it. On a scale from 0 to 6, none of the counsellors rated themselves at the extremes (i.e. totally directive or non-directive).

The degree of directiveness may vary according to the seriousness of the condition in question. In a recent European study a directive approach was adopted by many when the condition was lethal (e.g. anencephaly) or relatively minor (e.g. cleft lip). Non-directive approaches were related to late-onset disorders (e.g. Huntington's disease) and disorders with variable expression (e.g. sickle cell disease) (Marteau *et al.* 1994*b*).

These studies demonstrate clearly how the discussion on the directiveness of genetic counselling has so far taken a rather simplistic view of the issue and ignored the complexity of the flow of information and feelings that take place in the encounter between the counsellor and the counsellee.

In fact, non-directiveness itself as a goal may turn problematic. In an empirical study it was found that the more neutral the counsellor was perceived to be, the higher the counsellee perceived his or her own risk to be (Shiloh and Saxe 1989, cited by Michie *et al.* 1997*a*). One possible explanation was that, when the counsellor was perceived as non-directive, he or she was also perceived to be concealing bad news. In addition, directive counselling is no more effective than a non-directive approach in deterring high-risk couples from having children (*Lancet* 1982).

The idea of non-directive genetic counselling may be considered confusing by many parents who expect something else. The issue was addressed in a Finnish study on families having received genetic counselling between 1972 and 1981 (Somer *et al.* 1988). Firstly, 25% of the respondents stated that they had been encouraged to have more children and 2% felt the opposite. Secondly, when asked whether they wanted to hear only the facts or also the doctor's advice about having more children, 42% expressed a wish to hear both.

According to a British study, patients came to genetic counselling expecting information (79%), explanation (63%), reassurance (50%), advice (50%) and help in making decisions (30%) (Michie *et al.* 1997*b*). Thus a considerable degree of directiveness was expected by the counsellees in this study. In another study by the same group, none of the measures of directiveness was associated with counsellee satisfaction with information, mood, or the extent to which counsellee expectations were met (Michie *et al.* 1997*a*).

The clients may not be the only ones who are not happy with the idea of non-directive counselling. Some counsellors have expressed their awareness of a discrepancy between non-directiveness and the needs of the people they work with (White 1998). In addition, the expectation of unconditional support for the clients' decision – even if it is felt to be unethical – can be highly stressful for the counsellor (White 1998).

As already noted, genetic counsellors do not regard themselves as totally non-directive, although non-directiveness is a commonly shared ideal. Many studies have been done on the differences between counsellors in the degree of directiveness. Men have been shown to be more directive than women (Wertz and Fletcher 1988), obstetricians more directive than geneticists, and the latter more directive than genetic nurses (Marteau *et al.* 1994*a*). However, the extent to which these reported differences in attitude reflect 'real differences in practice rather than awareness of the "professionally correct" responses on questionnaires' is uncertain (Clarke 1997*b*, p. 184).

What people expect is, of course, very much related to social and cultural factors, and it reflects the general expectations they have towards health care personnel. The question of directiveness in genetic counselling can be seen as a part of a larger issue, namely paternalism in health care.

As with paternalism, it is far too simple to regard directiveness as a one-dimensional on-off phenomenon. The encounter between the doctor and the patient is so complex that genuine non-directiveness may be as unattainable as non-paternalism.

What is good genetic counselling?

Fully directive genetic counselling violates the autonomy of clients or patients in such a way that it is clearly unacceptable. Fully non-directive genetic counselling cannot be attained, and, even if it could be, the clients or patients would not necessarily be satisfied with it. They want a counsellor who has a set of values and is not a mere provider of information (Wertz 1997). This trend has even been noted in two national reports on genetic screening, one by the Nuffield Council and the other by the Danish Council, which mentioned moral counselling (Hoedemakers 1998).

Some professionals and lay advocacy groups have also criticised the notion of non-directiveness. Examples of the latter are some organised consumer groups that have said that professionals may tell consumers what they themselves would do if they were in the consumers' position (Wertz 1997). An example of the former is Seymour Kessler, a pioneer in training genetic counsellors, who in a 1996 meeting of the National Society of Genetic Counsellors pointed out that clients can be poorly served by mere provision of information in the absence of constructive help and guidance (Wertz 1997). He argued also that telling clients that you 'will support whatever decision they make' may actually be highly directive in that clients want to be able to say: 'I disagree with you. I am going to take my own course' (Wertz 1997).

Therefore, it has been suggested that we should avoid such problematic words altogether. For example, White (1998) suggested a reconfiguration of autonomy in the context of genetic counselling. She argues that autonomy has been interpreted as a negative right, the clients' right to non-interference in decision-making. Instead, it could be viewed as a positive right, the right to a maximally enhanced decision-making capacity.

White characterises her new approach as 'dialogical counselling'. The term dialogue is to be understood here broadly; it may involve conversing with another person, consulting an authoritative text or creating an internal debate. A dialogue requires at least two 'voices'.

In dialogical counselling the counsellors are responsible for ensuring that decisions are as fully informed and carefully deliberated as possible. The counselling procedure retains many of the features of the standard non-directiveness-oriented counselling. While the latter focuses on biomedical matters, the former focuses on clients' values, experiences and circumstances (White 1998). Counselling remains non-prescriptive, but it is possible for the counsellors to introduce unsolicited information or challenge what they believe are questionable choices (White 1998). Hoedemaekers (1998, p. 129) also called for a 'joint search for a morally excusable decision' and asked whether the individual autonomy and decision-making of (future) patients are really taken seriously if they are *not* confronted with (possibly) diverging views. Good genetic counselling does not take place in a moral or social vacuum. In White's words: ' "Good" decisions are defined as those that are fully informed and well reasoned, and in which client's goals, values and circumstances are optimally balanced – in a state of "reflective equilibrium" – with their moral and social implications' (White 1999, p. 20).

Geneticisation

In the beginning of this chapter genetic counselling was linked to medical conditions or diseases that are, or may be, genetic in origin. In today's world, it is worth reflecting for a while on the role of genes in our lives more generally. The following headlines are not uncommon: 'Cause of mental retardation is discovered' (*Financial Times* 22 March 1995). 'Alcoholism, over-eating and madness are inherited' (*Helsingin Sanomat* 8 November 1996; my translation). 'Genes reveal your destiny' (*Aamulehti* 4 May 1997; my translation). These are actual examples of a very common way of reporting news on scientific research on the human genome. The general formula of a news report for a finding is the following: 'It was announced today by scientists at (Harvard, Vanderbilt, Stanford) Medical School that a gene responsible for (some, many, a common form of) (schizophrenia, Alzheimer's, arteriosclerosis, prostate cancer) has been located and its DNA sequence determined. This exciting research, say scientists, is the first step in what may eventually turn out to be a possible cure for this disease' (Lewontin 1997, p. 29).

What was actually discovered in the first example? Not a general cause of mental retardation, of course, but mutations in a regulator gene, XH2, that are responsible for an extremely rare syndrome called ATR-X, which includes severe ID, anaemia, characteristic facial features and genital abnormalities. So far, about 50 individuals with the syndrome have been identified.

What did the second headline refer to? The text reports vaguely, and much more modestly, some findings concerning the role of genes in alcoholism, obesity and schizophrenia. Genes do not determine any of these conditions but increase susceptibility for them, it is concluded.

The third example taken was from a more general report on genetic research in a major Finnish newspaper. The article concentrated on the current state of genetic knowledge, and the text was more modest than the headline, which is common.

It is not only diseases that are stated to be genetically determined, but also traits like religiosity, political orientation, job satisfaction, leisure-time interests and proneness to divorce, according to a claim based on studies done on identical twins (Horgan 1993). There are selfish genes, pleasure-seeking genes, celebrity genes, gay genes, and the like (Nelkin and Lindee 1995). A recent report in the *Lancet* suggests that the bad behaviour of adolescents has a genetic basis (McGuffin and Tapar 1997). And, finally, a headline tells us that 'Faulty genes lead to old age' (cited by Spallone 1997), and in Minnesota a 1994 gubernatorial candidate from the religious right contended: 'There is a genetic predisposition for men to be heads of households' (cited by Nelkin and Lindee 1995, p. 107).

The preceding examples are recent, and it might appear that the idea of explaining almost everything in terms of genes is the result of the rapid development that has occurred in genetic technology in the past 20 years. However, already in 1907, Burbank (cited by Nelkin and Lindee 1995, p. 19) wrote the following words: 'Stored within heredity are all joys, sorrows, loves, hates, music, art, temples, palaces, pyramids, hovels, kings, queens, paupers, bards, prophets and philosophers . . . and all the mysteries of the universe.'

The common denominator of the examples is *geneticisation*, which refers to the 'ongoing process by which priority is given to searching for variations in DNA sequences that differentiate people from each other and to attributing some hereditary basis to most disorders, behaviours and physiological variations' (Lippman 1994, p. 13). The term has its roots in the concepts of scientisation and, more specifically, medicalisation (Parsons 1997).

Geneticisation can occur at different levels (Hoedemaekers 1998). Firstly, it can occur at the conceptual level, when genetic terminology is used to define problems (genes for violence, fatness, etc.). The second level is institutional and involves specific genetic expertise to deal with problems (e.g. the distribution of medical research funding). The third level at which geneticisation takes place is cultural, and genetic knowledge and technology lead to changing individual and social attitudes towards reproduction, health care, prevention and control of disease. Finally, the fourth level of geneticisation is philosophical in that genetic imagery may influence our views on human identity and individual responsibility (e.g. the limits of free will).

Geneticisation can be seen as the younger brother of the specific aetiology theory that flourished in the late nineteenth and early twentieth centuries. According to it, a necessary and sufficient cause can be found for most diseases. The success of the latter was obvious with the advent of medical microbiology and the popularity of the former relates to advances in molecular medicine.

The most obvious problem with geneticisation is that it oversimplifies extremely complex issues. A scientific *salto mortale* is performed in the drawing of conclusions on the basis of genetic findings and human behaviour, and the importance of the environment is ignored or underestimated.

Behind geneticisation

Why have genetic explanations become so popular? Scientific development has, of course, been faster than anyone could possibly foresee some decades ago, but this pace does not totally explain the current *genomania* (Lewontin's term). Other explanations can be found in general political development, the diminishing role of religion, the relative simplicity of genetic explanations, and the role of the media, especially science reporting.

Geneticisation implies a shift of responsibility from society to the individual in the sense that if, for example, alcoholism and crime are explained in terms of genes, no societal change can be hoped to be of any help. This shift aligns with the current political climate in many Western countries (Conrad 2001). Genetic explanations appear to provide a rational and neutral justification for existing social categories (Nelkin and Lindee 1995, p. 194).

Explicit religious metaphors referring to the genome as the Bible, the Holy Grail or the Book of Man are common, as are more secular metaphors like a map, a library or a recipe. Nelkin and Lindee (1995) have remarked that DNA has assumed a cultural meaning similar to that of the Biblical soul. Like the soul, DNA is invisible but real, and it is relevant to morality, personhood and social place. In a way it is even immortal. Thus the vacuum of the diminishing role of religion in Western societies has been partially filled by other issues.

Although the scientific issues in genetics are extremely complex and beyond comprehension for most people, the idea of 'one gene – one consequence' is attractive, when the alternatives are vague, incomplete and extremely complex social explanations. The expected specificity of genetic explanations raises hope for straightforward solutions or 'magic bullets' to alleviate human suffering (Conrad 1997, p. 142).

It is easy to blame irresponsible media for the exaggeration of the meaning of scientific results. Often the contents of the articles do not match the headlines, which report 'breakthroughs' and 'new hopes' (Kärki 1998). An analysis of genetics reporting in the *Helsingin Sanomat*, the largest newspaper in Finland, shows clearly a discrepancy between the headlines and the contents (Lauren 1998). A possibly unintended effect is that the public image of the role of genes is more deterministic than could be argued on the basis of the study results. It is not, however, only the journalists who create the news. Scientists have their role in writing their press releases, which form the basis of news reports. It was found in Lauren's survey that nine out of ten articles reporting found or localised genes were very optimistic about drugs or gene therapy that could soon be developed.

An illuminating example of the relationship between science and the media is the introduction of the term 'gay gene' into popular and scientific discourse (Conrad 2001). The first report relating homosexuality and a genetic marker was published in July 1993. Let me set aside the scientific issue itself and concentrate on how the finding was reported and what followed.

The report reached the front pages of most major newspapers in the USA (and probably elsewhere as well, although I am not aware of any research in this respect). The report explicitly noted that it is unlikely that a single gene would be responsible for homosexuality. However, several articles began, for the first time, to use the term 'gay gene' to describe the findings. Within the next two years the term became more common, and when Dean Hamer, the scientist behind the finding, and a journalist published a book about the research leading to the discovery, 'gay gene' appeared in the subtitle of the book.

A term like 'gay gene' is partially a journalistic short cut for a longer and scientifically more precise expression (e.g. a marker for a gene predisposing to homosexuality). At the same time, however, it probably indicates an increasing acceptance of the geneticisation of homosexuality. Of relevance is also the usage of the term: do we write about a gay gene, the gay gene or the 'gay gene'.

'Gay gene' is an example of 'the one gene issue', a tendency to oversimplify complex genetic issues. Another example of geneticisation in science reporting is 'the disconfirmation dilemma' (Conrad 2001). This phenomenon refers to the fact that new findings in genetic research are prominently reported in the news media, but findings that disconfirm or do not replicate earlier findings are far less frequently and prominently reported. This trend follows the logic of news: finding something new is news, but not finding it may not be (Conrad 2001). I shall return to the consequences of this disconfirmation dilemma later.

Consequences of geneticisation

Geneticisation does not only mean a minor side-track in the discourse on genetics and the philosophy of science. It has consequences that reach beyond these disciplines and involve science more generally, social life and even legal practice.

Geneticisation implies determinism and reductionism that, as such, are not new phenomena but have recurred in each generation since Darwin's day, argues Steven Rose (1995, p. 380). According to Rose, what is new is the way in which the mystique of the new genetics is seen as strengthening the reductionist argument.

Rose goes on to argue that naïve neurogenetic determinism is based on a faulty reductive sequence whose steps include: reification, arbitrary agglomeration, improper quantification, belief in statistical 'normality', spurious localisation, misplaced causality, and dichotomous partitioning between genetic and environmental causes.

Reification means that a dynamic process is converted into a static phenomenon. An example is violence, which is converted into a 'character', aggression. It can then be studied in isolation or as a part of the dynamically interactive system in which it appears.

The next step is arbitrary agglomeration, which lumps together many reified interactions as exemplars of one thing. I have already mentioned a recent report on the genetic basis of bad behaviour, which concludes with a suggestion that the bad behaviour of adolescents is probably heritable (McGuffin and Tapar 1997).

In improper quantification, numeric values are given to these reified and agglomerated characters. IQ is an example, and problems related to it have already been discussed in Chapter 2, as have the problems with the next step, statistical normality. Another example of problematic quantification is a gene for 'novelty seeking', which made headlines in early 1996. Two research reports in *Nature Genetics* suggested a causal relationship between the D4 dopamine receptor gene and the normal personality trait of novelty seeking (Benjamin *et al.* 1996, Ebstein *et al.* 1996). The studies were based on the hypothesis that novelty seeking is mediated by dopamine neurotransmission. Again, the validity of the findings is not the issue; instead I wish to make one remark concerning the significance of the results. In the latter study the effect size (i.e. the difference in questionnaire scores between groups with and without the particular allele) was 0.5 SD units. Statistical significance was, of course, reached but what does a difference of 0.5 SD units mean? In IQ it would be 7 or 8 points, in the birth weight of males with 40 weeks' gestation it is about 200 grammes. I cannot see that a difference of this magnitude would be particularly significant in a person's life.

Rose's next step, spurious localisation, refers to the way of speaking of, for example, gay or schizophrenic brains or genes rather than of brains or genes of a gay or schizophrenic person. As noted earlier, this is not only shorthand, but also reflects and perhaps endorses geneticisation and determinism. The latter extends, of course, beyond genes and genetics, an example being the localisation of gayness in the hypothalamus or corpus callosum.

Misplaced causality does not concern the relationship between genes and behaviour or disease, since the changes that take place in the genome of an individual during life cannot be attributed to behaviour, with the exception of some environmental exposures leading to DNA changes in particular tissues (e.g. smoking leading to lung cancer). With misplaced causality Rose refers to the problem of defining the direction of causality when a correlation between a brain structure or pattern of metabolism and a disease or particular type of behaviour is found.

The final step in this faulty reductive sequence is dichotomous partitioning between genetic and environmental causes. Cases in which the genotype of an individual determines the course of life are limited to rare single-gene defects like Huntington's disease. In the vast majority of cases, however, it is the interplay between genes and the environment that determines the lives of people. The 'genetic fatalism' that underlies much public discourse about genetics has expanded beyond scientific knowledge (Conrad 2001).

An obvious political consequence of geneticisation is that it turns attention away from the social and economic conditions that lead to violence, depression, obesity and the like, and also the environmental conditions that lead to diseases like cancer. If violence is explained in terms of one's genetic makeup, society is relieved of the collective responsibility that fosters violence (Nelkin and Lindee 1995). BRCA1 and BRCA2 genes are linked to breast cancer, but they account only for a small percentage of all cases. Genes predisposing to colon cancer have been located, but, again, they explain only a minor part of the total, dietary factors playing a major role in determining the incidence. It has been suggested that we could 'map' the environment for sources of 'susceptibility' instead of mapping the genome (Abby Lippman, cited by Harper and Clarke 1997, p. 104). As a consequence, in health research, there is the danger that important areas become neglected because tremendous costs and efforts are directed towards genetic research.

A consequence of the disconfirmation dilemma is that through the reporting of genetic discoveries, the discoveries are infused into the culture, while the neglect of disconfirmations produces 'errant cultural residues, obsolete ideas that remain part of public knowledge' (Conrad 2001).

Geneticisation may be manifest even in legal practice. Nelkin and Lindee (1995) have reported a custody dispute from 1990 in which a Californian couple had both donated their gametes and contracted with a surrogate to carry the fertilised egg to term. However, the surrogate mother refused to relinquish the baby at birth. The judge awarded sole custody to the couple but did not justify the decision by referring to the original contract. Instead, he linked the child's proper place to his genetic lineage and called the surrogate mother a 'genetic hereditary stranger' to the child.

One consequence of the exponential increase in genetic knowledge is that it may question our traditional views about responsibility and free will. Geneticisation considers genes as agents of destiny, and moral responsibility is removed from individuals by the biological excuse, hence the concept of 'genetic fatalism' (Nelkin and Lindee 1995, Conrad 2001). Currently, we are far from being able to determine how much of an action is genetically determined and how much is free will. Genetics may, however, call into question some traditional ideas about freedom and responsibility. As Parens (1996, p. 16) has noted, 'it may be that some of the dominant ways of thinking about those ideas have been simplistic and are no longer tenable'. If the idea of an absolutely free will has to be abandoned due to the results of genetic science, there is no need to throw away the concept of responsibility as well. And even if an IQ gene or genes were located some day, this finding would not dictate any social policy (Parens 1996).

Concluding remarks

The Nazi legacy and related fears of eugenic associations led to the development of genetic counselling more than half a century ago. In spite of the vigorous efforts to take distance from eugenic ideas, the tension still exists and will do so in the future. A logical connection prevails between genetic counselling and the incidence of genetic disease. By establishing a screening programme and related counselling services, society aims at reducing the incidence of the disease in question. Enhancing autonomy cannot serve as a primary goal, but it can instead form a condition that determines the means used for setting goals. In fact, the use of patient autonomy as the primary goal may turn into patient abandonment (Bosk 1992).

The same tension is reflected also in the difficulties found in measuring the success of genetic counselling. If the clients' decisions are as fully informed and carefully deliberated as possible, the success is maximal from the point of view of the clients and the counsellor. However, from a more general point of view there seem to be no good means with which to measure the success of genetic counselling.

The nature of the counselling process itself has varied with time, and today's practices show considerable variance between countries and individuals. Non-directiveness is an ill-defined ideal, and it is questionable whether it can or even should ever be attained. Good genetic counselling respects the autonomy of clients but considers also the moral and social implications of their decisions.

It is, of course, possible that some day more genes will be found that cause breast cancer, the role of genes predisposing to homosexual behaviour will be confirmed and the interaction between genes and environmental factors under certain conditions will be clarified. So far, however, the data are only fragmentary. With respect to, for example, violence, '*some* people may, under *some* environmental conditions, have a predisposition to violence in *some* circumstances *some* of the time' (Callahan 1996, p. 14). This situation is a long way from any specification, and it is hard to imagine a science that could predict whether such a predisposition would lead to violent behaviour in a particular place at a particular time. There is also a conceptual issue: how should we think about a person with a 'gay gene' who does not behave homosexually or of a person with a gene for alcoholism if he or she does not drink?

Advances in genetics have had a far greater impact on detection, diagnosis, screening, prevention and counselling than on therapy. Whatever is written in grant applications and press releases, there still remains a serious gap between disease characterisation and therapeutic utility (Friedmann 1990). As to prevention, the major solution so far has been the selective termination of affected pregnancies, and it is questionable whether this practice can be hailed as a great victory of modern science. Lewontin (1997, p. 52) goes as far as claiming that the use of genetic counselling and selective abortion is 'a sign, not of the success of molecular biology in producing a scientific medicine, but of its failure'.

The exaggerated hope molecular medicine has provided for people suffering from various inherited conditions was the subject of a recent editorial in *Thorax*. The editorial points out that the prognosis, for example, for cystic fibrosis patients, depends 'more upon the less glamorous development of current methods, and perhaps new pharmacological approaches, than upon gene therapy' (Dodge 1998, p. 158).

After all the criticism that has been presented here about geneticisation, it would not be fair not to recognise the great potential genetic science has to alleviate human suffering. The criticism against geneticisation comes partly from within genetic society and partly from outside groups, like philosophers and sociologists. Peter Conrad (1997) calls the latter to be active players in the discourse. Credibility is lost if it is denied that genes can have an effect on social behaviour. There is a role for social science in research into the interaction between genes and social structures. There is also a role for philosophy in clarifying conceptual issues, revealing value judgements and enquiring into the questions of empirical science.

How is all this relevant to my main issue, the prevention of ID? Since it is the commonest form of disability in children and genetic aetiology represents 30 to

50% of the cases, the consequences of geneticisation are highly relevant, at least in the following ways.

Firstly, geneticisation may overemphasise the role of genes in the development of ID, and the role of environmental factors may therefore be given less attention both in the public eye and in scientific discourse. This situation, in turn, would lead (or has already led) to the distortion of the balance in research resources. Secondly, geneticisation may raise unjustified hopes for gene therapy to correct errors leading to ID. The prenatal diagnosis of Down syndrome has been available for over three decades, but abortion remains the only option for prevention. Thirdly, the general fatalism associated with geneticisation may create a discouraging atmosphere in the education of intellectually disabled people, whatever the aetiology of the disability.

Since a great deal of intellectual disability is genetic in origin, the issues discussed in this section are actualised in the encounters between health professionals and lay people. But should ID always be prevented? And *why* should it be prevented? That is the topic of the next chapter.

Why should intellectual disability be prevented?

In the chapter on prevention I briefly discussed the general reasons that have been presented as a justification for the prevention of ID. This chapter examines each of the issues in detail. The arguments considered are (1) the eugenic argument, (2) the foetal-wastage argument, (3) the family burden argument, (4) the societal burden argument and (5) the quality of life argument.

But before going to the individual arguments something must be said about a common factor behind arguments 3, 4 and 5, namely, the issue of preventing *suffering*. With different stress, these arguments seem to take it for granted that ID causes suffering by the individual, the family or society. It is also assumed that this suffering should be avoided if possible. Behind these arguments seems to be the utilitarian idea that we are morally obliged to diminish or at least not increase the total sum of suffering in the world.

But what is suffering, and is it always an evil that should be avoided? Does ID *as such* always increase the amount of suffering in the world?

The word 'suffering' can mean a lot of things, 'from an absence of happiness to enduring extreme pain' (Hauerwas 1986, p. 30). Cassell (1995, p. 1899) has defined suffering as 'a specific state of severe distress induced by the loss of integrity, intactness, cohesiveness, or wholeness of the person, or by a threat that the person believes will result in the dissolution of his or her integrity'. Suffering is always individual, and it involves self-conflict. It has a *temporal* element in that there seems to be no suffering without the idea of a future (Cassell 1995).

Obviously, a conceptual distinction should be made between physical distress or pain and suffering. They overlap, but it is possible to be in pain without suffering and to suffer without pain. Essential to suffering is *meaning*, and sometimes suffering can be controlled merely by changing the meaning of the pain (Cassell 1995).

Is suffering always an evil that should be avoided? At least in some religious traditions suffering is not considered intrinsically wrong. Suffering may reveal a greater depth of human experience and meaning to the sufferer, and after the experience the person may also have a greater concern for the suffering of others

(Cassell 1995). But, of course, this is only afterwards, and it does not provide general justification for not preventing suffering.

In addition, a distinction can be made between suffering that merely happens and suffering that is a requisite for a goal. The former is more a matter of fate, and the latter a matter of choice, although the distinction may not always be so obvious (Hauerwas 1986).

Discussions about suffering in the case of an intellectually disabled child often do not specify the nature of suffering but, instead, remain vague. For example, Baby Doe's father (see Chapter 1), who had sometimes worked closely with Down syndrome children, was convinced that 'such children never had a minimally acceptable quality of life' (Kuhse and Singer 1985, p. 12). In a similar way a pregnant mother may say that she does not want to bring into this world a child that would inevitably suffer. Both seem to take it for granted that, for example, Down syndrome necessarily causes the person and the family to suffer. I shall return to the issue of quality of life later in this chapter and to Down syndrome in later chapters, but it is worth noting here that many families consider the suffering caused by the selective termination of a foetus with Down syndrome greater than the suffering caused by the birth of such a child.

John Harris' starting point in his treatise on the morality of selective termination is that it is wrong to bring avoidable suffering into the world, but he does not explain what he means by suffering (Harris 1998*b*). Neither does he consider the details of the alternatives (e.g. the actual life of a family with a Down syndrome child). The total amount of happiness may be beyond quantification, but, even if it would be possible to measure and compare the 'happiness units', it is not at all obvious that the selective termination option would win. Thus the situation is not so clear even inside the utilitarian framework.

Suffering from having an intellectually disabled child resembles the suffering of parents who are childless against their own wishes. In both cases the cause of suffering is *a lost chance*. Childless parents have lost the chance to see the growth and development of their own offspring. Parents with an intellectually disabled child have lost the chance to see their child develop like the majority of children do. Depending on the severity of the disability, they will perhaps not see their child become independent, marry, have their own children, and so forth. Instead, they will witness slow or prolonged development with an upper limit caused by the condition behind the disability. This suffering is related to the view we have of man and life: ' "retardation" might not "exist" in a society which values cooperation more than competition and ambition' (Hauerwas 1986, p. 161).

Of course, the condition behind disability may also cause physical pain either by itself or through procedures (like shunt operations) that are needed. Physical pain is not, however, the central issue in the context of suffering from being intellectually disabled or having an intellectually disabled child. If it would be, eliminating it would be a solution, and prevention would lose its meaning.

Eugenic argument

Eugenics has already been dealt with in the chapters concerning prevention and prenatal diagnosis. It was concluded that (1) the public health genetics of today can be defined as a form of eugenics, if the latter is understood as deliberate control of the perpetuation of human traits by social pressure, and (2) the application of prenatal diagnosis and selective abortion is *dysgenic*, not *eugenic*, when the total effect on the human gene pool is considered. The magnitude of this dysgenic effect is, however, very small.

The eugenic argument can be formulated as follows. A normal or healthy human genome can be exactly or approximately defined. There is something bad or undesirable in certain genetic conditions that deviate from this norm. The elimination of these conditions, defined as 'genetic diseases', can be considered a legitimate goal.

The eugenic argument assumes thus that 'genetically normal' or 'genetically healthy' can be defined. As we have seen in the chapter on the definition of ID, the concept of 'normal' is highly ambiguous.

A naturalistic view on health and disease equates the normal with the natural (e.g. Boorse 1975). It seems to assume that a species norm for a genotype can be identified. However, with the exception of identical twins, we all have unique genotypes, and it is a matter of convention which of them is considered normal and which abnormal or undesirable. In fact, virtually every one of us carries a small number of deleterious recessive genes and is, in Paul Ramsey's words, a 'fellow mutant' (Boss 1993, p. 156).

In addition, the interaction between one's genotype and the environment is, in many cases, a crucial determinant of health and well-being. A gene for sickle-cell anaemia was once advantageous in protecting from malaria; in present-day America it is no longer so.

As Canguilhem (1978, p. 138) noted, strictly speaking 'there is no biological science of the normal'. Physiology, for example, is a science of biological situations and conditions *called* normal. This normal is a polemical concept that 'negatively qualifies the sector of the given which does not enter into its extension while it depends on its comprehension' (Canguilhem 1978, p. 146). It refers to a *norm* which 'draws its meaning, function, and value from the fact of the existence, outside itself, of what does not meet the requirement it serves' (Canguilhem 1978, p. 146).

'Genetically healthy' is also a vague concept. It would seem to refer to a person whose 'total genetic make-up ... is such that it predisposes to and effectuates a state of perfect physical and mental health, perfect adaptational capacities in the individual, in the present as well as later in life, and that it does not contribute to genetically based health risks in future children' (Hoedemaekers 1998, p. 89). The meaningfulness of such a concept is questionable, because it isolates the individual from the environment and also from history, being thus an example of geneticisation (see Chapter 3). Even if we knew the complete genetic profile of a person, we would have very limited information about his or her health. Knowledge about gene–environment interaction would add something to this situation, but we would always have a far from complete picture of the role genes and gene–environment interaction play during the whole life-span of the individual in different environments.

The eugenic argument could also refer to the genetic health of a population or human species in general. This is not a very helpful concept either, since it is hopelessly narrow and reductionistic. Populations live in very different environments and conditions, and it is hardly possible to say that population A is genetically healthier than population B.

The eugenic argument is essentially utilitarian. References to the good of future generations carry the utilitarian message of the greatest good for the greatest number. Sometimes this message is clear, as in an editorial in the *Canadian Medical Association Journal* in 1927: 'How long will it be before we recognise that our children, too, have a right to be free; free from a heritage which weakens their minds or cripples their bodies' (cited by Cairney 1996, p. 791). Sometimes, especially in the Nazi doctrine, reference is made to a less clear good, that of a larger whole: 'Individualism as a basis for medical practice has been recognised as a false path. The patient is not an individual with particular demands; he is only one part of a much larger whole or unity: of his family, his race, his *Volk*' (Professor Verschuer in 1934, cited by Hubbard 1986, p. 233).

No science can provide complete answers to questions such as when does a deviation from the common gene constitute a genetic disease and when is it merely an interesting variation (Schwartz 1996). A 'normal' or 'standard' human genome will never be discovered, but it may be invented. To describe this standard then as the master race is an obvious consequence (Schwartz 1996), and the idea of the *Volk* would be there again.

Could the gene pool have some intrinsic value in itself? Or could perhaps some characteristic of it, like variety, have intrinsic value? Answers to these questions depend on the way we answer to the question of the value of nature in general: is it valuable in itself or only for living and future people? This, of course, is a major unsettled philosophical issue that cannot be addressed here. Some pragmatic remarks can, however, be made.

The influence of human activity on the (human) gene pool will be minute in the foreseeable future. As has been mentioned earlier, the total effect of prenatal diagnosis and screening may be dysgenic in the sense that the relative number of carriers of recessive genes leading to certain diseases may increase, while the homozygotes would be selectively aborted. This possibility shows the vagueness of the discussion: a favourable development in the health of the population may not necessarily correlate with changes in the gene pool of that population.

If human activity would some day result in less variety in the (human) gene pool and this lost variety were related to diseases overcome, the result could hardly be seen as bad development (assuming that no force would be used to achieve the change). The setting changes dramatically if the variety lost goes beyond genes related to diseases (Chadwick *et al.* 1998).

The power of the eugenic argument depends thus on how various terms are understood and how the good of an individual is weighed against the good of the community. The latter can be further understood as the present community or some hypothetical future community. The argument is powerful only if agreement can be reached concerning (1) which conditions are serious enough to allow preventive measures at the population level and (2) the balance between the interests of the individual (e.g. autonomy) and the community (e.g. economics). The issue is thus very much the same as in the discussion concerning the public health argument and the reproductive autonomy argument (see Chapter 5).

Foetal-wastage argument

A great majority of all conceptions never survive to birth. Close to two-thirds of all pregnant women lose their embryos during the first trimester and more miscarry during the latter two trimesters. The frequency of chromosomal aberrations among these spontaneously aborted embryos or foetuses is far higher than among live-born babies. According to the foetal-wastage argument, induced selective abortion is simply a continuation of this natural process (Boss 1993). Leon Kass (1985, p. 96) thinks that 'This standard, . . . is one that most physicians and genetic counsellors appeal to in their heart of hearts, no matter what they say or do about letting the parents choose'. In fact, the argument has also been used to support abortion in general: 'If Nature resorts to abortion to maintain genetic stability by discarding as many as 3 in every 4 conceptions, it will be difficult for anti-abortionists to oppose abortion on moral or ethical grounds' (Roberts and Lowe 1975, cited by Murphy 1985).

Behind the argument there seem to be two assumptions. Firstly, nature seems to be able to differentiate between embryos or foetuses that have the possibility for full human life after birth and those that do not. Secondly, nature or natural is considered the standard from which we can infer how things should be.

The first assumption is partly true. It is not true, however, that the more serious (from our point of view) a condition is, the more frequently spontaneous abortions occur. Turner syndrome (45, X) is usually considered to be a relatively mild condition. Modern hormone replacement therapy leads to normal pubertal development for girls with this syndrome, leaving relatively short stature and infertility as the only characteristics to indicate the lack of an X chromosome. Today, even infertility can be overcome with donated eggs. On the other hand, Edwards syndrome (trisomy 18) is a very serious condition with defects in multiple organs and death shortly after birth. Yet the proportion of Turner syndrome embryos and foetuses which spontaneously abort is apparently much higher that the respective proportion with Edwards syndrome. Even if we consider ourselves as successors of the work of nature, the latter's view on the seriousness of conditions would be in conflict with our common sense.

In addition, from an evolutionary point of view, nature works in ways that do not necessarily eliminate genotypes that decrease mental or intellectual fitness. Fragile X syndrome is a common genetic disorder causing ID in males while the heterozygous women have no or only mild symptoms. However, there is direct evidence of increased reproductive success among these women (Nesse and Williams 1994). The PKU gene seems to reduce the likelihood of miscarriage and perpetuate itself despite causing disease (Nesse and Williams 1994). If some genes increase the susceptibility for schizophrenia, these same genes are probably also advantageous in combination with certain other genes or in certain environments (Nesse and Williams 1994).

A more severe problem with the foetal-wastage argument, however, is the second assumption, according to which what happens in nature is good as such and the goal of medicine should be, at least in this respect, to enhance a natural process. The assumption raises questions about the relationship between nature and morals and also between nature and medicine.

'Nature' and 'natural' have been used with very many meanings. To cite Leon Kass (1996, p. 22) concerning our intellectual confusion about what nature truly is:

Whose nature do we wish to bring to the aid of ethics: the nature of Aristotle (purposive) or Lucretius (atomist and hedonic) of Seneca (rationally lawful) or Descartes (rationalistically mathematical) or Hobbes (passionate and dangerous) or Rousseau (bountiful and self-lovingly free) or Darwin (historical and competitive) or Nietzsche (will to power) or Whitehead (thoroughly organic)?

Today, in our culture, nature primarily has one of four possible meanings. Firstly, nature can be understood as everything that there is or that takes place in the physical world of experience (Karjalainen and Häyry 1992, Honderich 1995). To be natural is to be part of nature. We humans are nothing special although we may differ from other animals because of our cognitive abilities. For those who think that nothing exists outside nature (supernatural, the Creator, God, etc.), there cannot be anything non-natural (i.e. whatever we humans do is by definition natural). Those who think that there is something outside nature must consider man's role in relation to nature and the supernatural. These issues are, of course, beyond the scope of this book, but the question remains of whether nature, as God's Creation or not, is necessarily good.

Secondly, nature can be understood as the living world as opposed to the non-living. Many philosophical problems follow (e.g. of definition or demarcation). From our point of view the question of the goodness of nature is similar to the one already presented.

Thirdly, nature, and especially the organic world, can be set off against humans and the consequences of their work. Natural is everything that happens independently of human activity or is subconscious human activity. This view, too, leaves open the question of whether nature is good as such or only inasmuch it has been altered and cultivated by humans.

Fourthly, nature (or Nature) can be understood as a subject: it takes revenge if you do wrong. This type of view is common in some original cultures but it is also often referred to in our cultures as an argument to support, for example, some alternative forms of medicine. (The concept of alternative medicine is far from clear, and there is a large grey area between conventional or school medicine and alternative or complementary medicine.) The only way to find out what is wrong, however, is to act, wait and see. If a disaster follows in one form or another, we have acted unnaturally. It is obvious that this view of nature fails to help us in deciding exactly how we have to act in particular situations.

Whether nature can ever help us with moral issues is, of course, a large philosophical question, and it cannot be settled here. The tradition of natural law or naturalism is old in philosophy, but there has hardly been a philosopher who has claimed that nature is *necessarily* good. Whether G. E. Moore was right or wrong in stating that 'good' is necessarily a 'non-natural' quality is still debated. Today there is at least one field of inquiry and action, environmentalism, in which nature is considered the standard for proper behaviour (Callahan 1996).

The supporters of the foetal-wastage argument seem to assume that nature is good, at least with respect to this particular issue of spontaneous abortions. This conclusion does not, however, follow directly from any of the four formulations of what nature is. And even if we accepted that nature serves as a moral guide in this issue, there is no obvious reason why we should stop here. Why not enhance other natural processes in which beings that are considered not able to lead a 'full and independent' life are abandoned or destroyed? What other phenomena in nature are good as such, and what could be the distinctive criteria for something to be considered good? Exactly when is it good to interfere in the processes of nature?

Another problem with the second assumption behind the foetal-wastage argument concerns the relationship between nature and medicine. If we see ourselves just as a part of nature, then everything we do, also in medicine, is natural, independently of the question of whether it is right or wrong. If we see ourselves as having a distinctive position, then our medicine is, by definition, *interfering* with nature. In most cases medicine in fact somehow interferes with the natural way things go, unless, for example, in terminal care we let 'nature take its course'.

This interference can take place in several ways. Sometimes medical intervention acts *against* natural processes (like antibiotics), and sometimes it *enhances* natural processes (like thyroid hormone replacement in hypothyreosis). The aim is to *restore* a state (as in the treatment of an infection) or to *make possible* a state (as in the treatment of congenital hypothyreosis) or to *alleviate* symptoms. The enhancement of natural processes can take place at the individual level (hormone replacement) or at a communal level (adding iodine to salt), where individuals benefiting from the procedure cannot be specified. Selective abortion could also be seen as an enhancement process, but not in the same sense, since what is enhanced is an ill-defined and inconsistent 'principle' of nature taking place during early pregnancy.

It seems obvious to me that the foetal-wastage argument, at least in its present form, is weak and cannot provide justification for the prevention of intellectual disability. The general idea of everything in nature being good would lead to odd implications, and the particular idea of certain spontaneous abortions being good leads us to ask why this and not some other natural process should be considered good. It may be that the supporters of the argument base their view on a value judgement about the lives of individuals with a certain genotype or phenotype. This question will be addressed in the following chapter. But before that, I still have three arguments to deal with.

Family burden argument

The family burden argument can be presented in two forms, as a more general version referring to rights and as a narrower utilitarian version comparing the family consequences of accepting a handicapped child or aborting it as a foetus. According to the general version, parents have the right to determine both the qualitative and the quantitative character of their families (Kass 1985). This stance is similar to the standard liberal argument for abortion. In the context of ID the narrower formulation is, however, commoner. Accordingly, if the parents believe that the birth of a child with certain characteristics will cause suffering and sorrow to themselves and to their other children and drain their time and resources, they have the right to prevent the birth.

Below I first consider the utilitarian version of the argument. In the latter part of this chapter I deal more generally with the issue of parental choice of, for example, the sex of an offspring. It may be worth noting that the prenatal technology needed to examine the characteristics of the foetus is available only to a minority of the world's families. In many developing countries it is available only to a very small minority who can afford it, and the major reason for its introduction may have been sex selection, not the prevention of physical or intellectual handicaps.

Depending on the degree of the disability and the number of additional handicaps, the burden an intellectually disabled child lays on a family can be anything from minute to substantial. The discovery of disability in a child of any age is always a shock, but a mildly intellectually disabled child with no additional handicaps may later bring only minor changes to family life. On the other hand, the care of a severely intellectually disabled child with, for example, cerebral palsy and epilepsy may be extremely time consuming and exhausting, both physically and mentally.

No doubt, an intellectually disabled child always brings about a crisis in a family, but the impact is not entirely and straightforwardly negative. There are both families that have been weakened and families that report to have been emotionally enriched by the presence of a disabled child. It is important to note that the matter in each case is *uncertain* and the experience may strengthen as well as weaken the family. And, of course, as Bosk (1992, p. 56) has pointed out, 'chronic sorrow' and 'successful normalisation' are only analytically distinct. Empirically, it is possible to imagine the same person having each feeling closely connected in time.

The burden on the family is, to a large extent, a culturally determined construct and cannot be separated from the social structure of society. Health care arrangements (private or public), mothers' work outside the home and the infrastructure of services for the intellectually disabled are some important factors contributing to family well-being. While in the USA the hardship experienced by families with an intellectually disabled child is largely determined by economic factors, only a relatively small percentage of families in Northern Ireland feel that they cannot accomplish a viable marital relationship, a satisfying parental relationship or their basic aims in life (Burton 1975 cited in Boss 1993).

The burden on the family is expressed in several ways. Firstly, having an intellectually disabled child is an obvious risk for both the marriage and the relationships between the parents and the other children in the family. Secondly, whatever the arrangements of care, the parents often experience feelings of guilt. They may feel guilty of the mere fact that they have brought a handicapped child into this world or they may feel guilty of placing the child in an institution. Thirdly, the burden on the family is expressed materially, as extra economic costs caused by the special care arrangements needed for the child.

Much empirical research has been done during the past few decades to explore well-being in families with intellectually disabled or otherwise handicapped children. The lives of families with a child with Down syndrome are discussed in Chapter 9, and I shall summarise here only the results of a recent, large Finnish study that examined the lives of 647 families with an intellectually disabled child (Itälinna *et al.* 1994).

- Most families managed to get along with the care of the child without large problems. A quarter felt only minor stress; on the other hand a quarter also felt major stress.
- Parents' pessimism and worries about the future of the child increased as the child grew older.
- With a few exceptions, parents' stress correlated with the degree of the child's disability.
- Parents' stress correlated with the quality of their relationship with each other.
- If there were other children in the family, the parents were less worried about the future of their intellectually disabled child.
- The amount of unofficial help from friends and relatives was small but very important.
- A majority of parents felt that parenting an intellectually disabled child had brought several positive things into their lives.

The amount of guilt parents feel after either aborting or accepting a child with ID may be substantial and long lasting. It is obviously very strongly related to both the psychological characteristics of the parents and the support provided by the health care system and society. Because parents often feel guilty *whatever* they choose, the result does not serve as support of the family burden argument – neither does it refute it.

The economic load on the family can be enormous, especially in countries like the USA and in families with incomplete insurance coverage. It has been estimated that 70% of families with a chronically disabled child in the USA have significant financial problems as a result of the child's disorder (Boss 1993). Many of the costs are hidden (i.e. days lost from work, special diets, travel costs, etc.). In countries where medical care is subsidised, the situation is different, and the economic burden on families is far less important.

We can conclude that the psychological and economic burden on families with an intellectually disabled child varies substantially and cannot be dealt with in vacuum, without the structure of society and, particularly the supportive services provided for these families being considered. Thus the utilitarian argument has not proved to be *generally* true. It is a good argument only in *particular* cases, in which the burden of a handicapped child on the family can reasonably be expected to exceed the burden caused by abortion.

Parental autonomy

The more general version of the familial burden argument claims that parents have the right to determine both the qualitative and the quantitative character of their families. Strong support for parental involvement comes from the fact that it is the parents who live with the child 24 hours a day for maybe years or decades, depending on the severity of the physical condition. It is the parents who concretely bear the psychological and, in many cases, economic burden.

One key issue is the question about the *limits* of parental autonomy. If, namely, only the parents are to decide what qualities they accept in their children, then we have to consider at least two kinds of difficult cases: the case of undesired sex and the case of deliberately accepting an abnormal child.

Sex selection

John Harris, arguing from a mostly utilitarian point of view, does not consider the issue of sex selection problematic: 'Either such traits as hair colour, eye colour, gender and the like are important or they are not. If they are not important why not let people choose? And if they are important, can it be right to leave such important matters to chance?' (Harris 1998*a*, p. 191). He also reminds that 'having a preference for producing a child of a particular gender by no means necessarily implies discrimination against the alternate gender any more perhaps that choosing to marry a co-religionist, a compatriot, or someone of the same race or even class implies discrimination against other religions, nations, races, or classes' (Harris 1998*a*, p. 192–3). A prerequisite for this kind of thinking is, of course, that abortion on demand is accepted up to the gestational age where the determination of sex is possible.

Harris does not deal with sex selection in relation to any particular society. It may, however, be illuminating to do so. Prenatal diagnosis for the determination of sex is only a common practice, for example, in India. The country is afflicted with the 'son-syndrome', and the birth of a female child, especially if she is not the first, is a calamity (Kusum 1993). A son will continue the name of the family and take care of the parents in their old age. According to the Hindu religion, a sonless father cannot achieve salvation. A daughter, on the other hand, is a constant burden to her parents, and a woman who has only daughters has to bear social embarrassment and even family harassment (Kusum 1993). A traditional solution to the problem has been female infanticide, which still takes place and is even supported by some doctors.

Prenatal determination of foetal sex began in India in the mid 1970s and soon became a flourishing business. For example, in 1987–1988 some 50 000 sex determination tests were recorded in Bombay only. Of the 8000 abortions preceded by amniocentesis in six Bombay hospitals in 1986, 7999 were female foetuses (Kusum 1993). After many years of heated discussion and campaigns a bill banning the selective abortion of female foetuses was passed in 1994 (Imam 1994). Later reports show, however, that, in spite of educational and economic improvements, the practice continues (Khanna 1997, Nielsen *et al.* 1997).

Five arguments to support prenatal diagnosis purely for sex determination have been presented in the Indian discussion (Kusum 1993).

Firstly, it has been argued that the status of females will improve when their number diminishes. This argument resembles the one presented in the context of ID: if, through selective abortion, there will be fewer intellectually disabled people, those surviving will be better off since they will have more resources. Both arguments are peculiar. The first seems to assume a turning point at which the disrespect of females turns to respect. How far should they go in India and should the government adopt this as an official policy to improve the status of women? The similar argument about the status of the intellectually disabled also makes a wild assumption of the use of certain resources only for them. Taken to an extreme, if various programmes for the prevention of ID were highly successful, the last intellectually disabled person on earth would be really well off.

Secondly, the practice has been supported as a family planning measure. Without it couples desiring to have a son would go on trying and having daughters, thus adding to the family size. While it may be true that the size of many families is smaller because of the availability of the practice, it is, however, a *side effect*, not the primary motivation for families. Accepting this argument also sends the message that the underlying discriminatory attitudes against women are accepted because of favourable side effects.

Thirdly, the argument has been presented that women should be left the final choice of the fate of their foetuses. Because women are entitled to a *general* right to decide about their pregnancies, choosing termination on the basis of the sex of the foetus should have no special position. In the Indian context, however, the argument turns into a farce, when women do not enjoy freedom 'even in the most intimate matters of their life' (Kusum 1993, p. 155). This argument resembles closely the one that has been put forward in the developed countries to justify selective abortion. It is the strongest argument for the practice and I shall return to it later.

Fourthly, it has been argued that banning sex determination tests would lead to widespread underhand practices with apparent dangers to the lives and health of women. This stand, again, is similar to the argument that has been used to justify the legalisation of abortion. Both arguments are, however, weak because they speculate something that will not *necessarily* happen. Their form is also so general that, with similar arguments, one could justify almost anything, like 'we should legalise drugs because banning them will inevitably lead to crime and misery'.

The fifth argument is related to the fourth one and states that the law would not be a very effective instrument to bring about change in the social attitudes of people. Although presented by Kusum (1993) as an argument of the protagonists, this is not really an argument to support the practice but a pragmatic statement about the relation of law and practice.

The first argument against prenatal sex selection is based on the unbalanced sex ratio that would follow, or has in fact been reported already in India. A fear has been expressed that, if the number of females continues to fall, there will be an increase in crimes like rape and incest, and the reproductive burden of women will increase. As has already been stated, however, the exact opposite was speculated to *support* the practice. It could as well be speculated that the imbalance would, in the future, lead to selective abortions performed on *male* foetuses. On a more theoretical level, it is not obvious that the ratio between the number of males and females has any intrinsic value.

The second argument against the practice refers to the health hazard it creates for women who cannot bear the hazards of the repeated test–abortion–test cycle. But what would be the alternative? With the current social attitudes a woman with repeated pregnancies without testing risks her health *even more* than the one who chooses testing.

The third argument against prenatal sex selection states simply that it is against the law. This is, of course, a valid argument only for those who agree with the law.

To conclude, most of the arguments presented either for or against the practice are not convincing. The third argument in support of the practice is, however, a strong one. If abortion is accepted as a *general* right of women, then there are no good reasons to demand justification in particular cases. In fact, in countries where girls are not wanted for cultural reasons, parents can refer also to the suffering the child herself will face if she survives. If we in the West wish to give parents a wide autonomy to decide about their offspring, we cannot justify our resentment about sex selection in a developing country. This is not, of course, to say that the situation in India, for example, is satisfactory and should be accepted. What I wish to argue is that a general concern about women's position is highly justified, but an isolated concern about the practice of sex selection is not necessarily that.

A duty to abort?

What about cases in which a woman or a couple deliberately accepts a child with a physical or intellectual handicap? John Harris, for example, has argued in this context that it can also be wrong not to terminate a pregnancy (Harris 1998*a*). He writes in a general way about 'bringing avoidable suffering into the world' and does not deal with details of handicaps or syndromes. He admits that behind his argument there is the assumption that replaceability is unproblematic. The issue of replaceability has been discussed widely in bioethics and accepted by many utilitarian philosophers (e.g. Parfit, Harris, Kuhse and Singer) since Hare brought it up in the 1970s (Hare 1976).

The main idea is that 'the next child in the queue', that is, the (probably healthy) child that would be born if the present defective foetus or infant were not in its way, may have important interests that overcome the interests of actual foetuses or infants. The next child in the queue is an example of 'possible people', who will exist if we act one way, but who will not exist if we act another way (Parfit 1976). Hare presents a case in which the interests of a foetus with an abnormality and a possible child of the same parents, Andrew, are compared. Andrew would be born later, if a handicapped child were not in his way. Hare does not specify the nature of the abnormality: 'I am deliberately not specifying any particular medical condition, because if I do I shall get my facts wrong' (Hare 1976, p. 366). Because Andrew has 'a high prospect of a normal and happy life' (Hare 1976, p. 369), the harm that would be done to him by stopping him from being conceived and born would be much greater than that done to a foetus or unsuccessfully operated newborn by killing it. (Hare is somewhat unclear here; he seems to refer to some surgical condition, possibly something like spina bifida, although he declined to specify the medical condition earlier.) In short, Hare presents a utilitarian argument: when the death of a disabled foetus or infant will lead to the birth of another infant with better prospects of a happy life, the total amount of happiness will be greater if the former is killed.

The replaceability argument is probably counterintuitive for most people, but it can also be shown to be severely insufficient for many rational reasons.

Firstly, I have discussed the replaceability argument so far only in the context of physical or intellectual disability. There is, however, no logical reason to limit the argument to such cases. To show the arbitrariness of the argument, let us look at a family living in a poor developing country. They are expecting their third child, and the prospects for the child will be poor in many respects. The woman has been told, that due to a uterine malformation, she will not be able to have more children than three. For some reason the family will be able to move to a developed country, and their life will be wealthier and more secure in many ways. This move will not, however, be possible for the next two years. The present pregnancy is at an early stage and could be terminated without seriously risking the woman's possibility to carry another pregnancy to term. According to the replaceability argument we should consider the rights of the 'next child in the queue' (i.e. the possible child to be born in the new country). Would Hare, Harris and other supporters of the replaceability argument demand that this pregnancy be terminated in the interests of the possible child who would be born in the new country?

Secondly, what would be the position of newborns with a known condition leading to ID or physical disability? At least Kuhse and Singer, who support the argument, also support infanticide in cases in which the newborn baby is severely handicapped. Because it is not a person, it does not have a right to live and is therefore morally in the same category as foetuses. Let us imagine again a family, this time one with a newborn child with Down syndrome. Since Kuhse and Singer think that the prospects of this child having a happy life would be poorer than those of a child with normal chromosomes, it would again be logical for them to suggest the killing of this child in the interests of a possible child to be born into this family later.

Thirdly, the proponents of the replaceability argument ignore totally the emotional crisis, which the abortion of a defective foetus brings about. The intensity of the crisis varies from minor to major. Barbara Katz Rothman, the author of *The Tentative Pregnancy*, tells an example of the latter:

> She had had her abortion and gone right back to work. She was a physician, as a matter of fact. And then one afternoon a couple of weeks later, she couldn't take it any more. She just started crying out of nowhere. Leaving the office and walking for hours, she found herself wandering in a bookstore at one point and, oddly enough, found my book. Standing in the store, she cried, recognizing herself and her grief in these women. She took a couple of months off, allowed herself time to recover from her loss, allowed herself time to understand her loss as real, genuine, and worthy of grief rather than purely of gratitude. (Rothman 1994, p. 269)

Fourthly, although, for example, Harris admits that replacing a foetus that will be disabled with one that will not be disabled may not be unproblematic, he gives the impression that a woman should have particularly good reasons not to have a termination in such cases. I respond by citing a young woman who has an intellectually disabled brother with fragile X syndrome and is now pregnant. Her brother's general intellectual level resembles that of a 5- or 6-year-old child. He cannot read or write but he is good at cooking and baking. Being a carrier of the syndrome, she had a DNA test during her first pregnancy. The male foetus did not have the fragile X syndrome. In a television interview a few years later, now also a mother of a girl, she was asked whether she would have chosen abortion if the first test would have shown the syndrome. She replied:

> Well, now I feel that, no, I would not have. And I also had the feeling then that I would not necessarily want an abortion. I had already had one miscarriage before my first pregnancy; also it frightened me in the beginning. I didn't necessarily agree with my husband, but he said that we would look at the situation after the tests. If it looked as if the child would be intellectually disabled, we would look and think carefully about it. I agreed with him that we should carefully think about what we would do, but, at that stage I was so emotionally involved that I couldn't have had an abortion. I had my brother and I had cared for him. Therefore, I didn't feel it would be as terrible a burden as my husband thought it might be. (My translation of a transcription from the programme *Human factor* in TV2 Finland, 25 April 1998)

This narrative reveals how complex the whole situation is and how crudely the idea of replacement simplifies the issue. Moral judgements are made on the grounds of abstract concepts like personhood, possible people or replaceability and particular contexts, in which decisions are made, are ignored or inadequately considered

(Vehmas 1999*a*, 1999*b*). We saw, for example, that Hare deliberately did not specify the medical condition. That creates a problem because, in real life, the foetus or the infant has a history, a family and a diagnosis, *all* of which are highly relevant to the moral judgements about its life. In Rayna Rapp's words: 'It matters whether one is African-American, Polish- or Irish Catholic, middle-class or working class or working-poor. But it also matters whether this is a first or a fourth pregnancy, whether you have experienced difficulties in becoming and staying pregnant, whether you had a cousin with Down or a neighbor who had hemophilia' (Rapp 1994, p. 229).

Fifthly, ID is still a special case. While we can assume that many syndromes or conditions causing gross physical handicaps certainly bring about suffering, this is not so with conditions causing only ID. I shall return to the quality of life issues in more detail later, but here it is important to note that, if an intellectually disabled person suffers from the disability per se, the suffering could be mediated through the meaning that his or her *environment* has given to the disability.

To conclude, parental autonomy has become an important value in many Western societies, and at the same time liberal abortion policies have been introduced in these societies. If abortion on request is generally accepted, I do not find any convincing arguments against prenatal sex determination. In addition, if parental autonomy is respected, it should also include the possibility to bring a physically or intellectually handicapped child deliberately into this world.

Societal burden argument

According to the societal burden argument, the intellectually disabled never become productive or otherwise benefit society. Instead, they are a burden, and, therefore, preventing states leading to ID and births of foetuses with conditions leading to ID is justified, if that prevention does not bring about a greater burden in one or another form.

It is obvious that the group is very heterogeneous with respect to productivity, but, excluding the mildest cases, it is certainly true that material productivity will never exceed the costs of the care these people need. Generally, the unit of measurement in the discussions on social burdens is money, other social burdens or goods being far more difficult to quantify.

Cost–benefit analyses

Monetary costs can (often) be measured and compared, and, therefore, it is understandable that money has been the unit of measurement in numerous cost–benefit analyses concerning the prevention of ID. Such analyses have been performed since the 1970s, and the screening for disorders like Down syndrome and fragile X syndrome has been shown to be cost-effective in several studies. These kinds of analyses are, however, problematic in many ways.

Firstly, the accuracy of the calculations can be questioned. Many assumptions must be made about, for example, the uptake of tests and the proportion of women willing to abort after a positive diagnosis. Even more difficult to estimate than screening-related costs are probably the costs to society for caring for the intellectually disabled in question. It is obvious, for example, that a person who is never able to work creates considerable costs for society. On the other hand, there are programmes and legislation that attempt to enable persons with handicaps to function like other people, be employed and be self-sufficient. The recent trend to close massive institutions and integrate the intellectually disabled into society probably also decreases the economic burden. In addition, most of the disorders leading to ID are extremely variable in their expression.

The validity of the calculations is further confounded by the great variance in the status of intellectually disabled people in society. For example, in Finland, it was practically a rule in the 1950s and early 1960s that a baby with Down syndrome was placed in an institution. Nowadays there are no children with Down syndrome in institutions, the great majority living in their own homes. Those few who are abandoned by their parents are cared for in foster homes. Thus the economic burden to society during the childhood years is substantially smaller than during the years of early institutionalisation.

Secondly, not all costs have been considered in the calculations. While it is often said that a normal child will replace an aborted defective child, costs or benefits related to this replacement have not been taken into account. What is even more important, the costs and benefits related to the unavoidable miscarriages related to amniocentesis have not been considered. If the saved lifetime costs of an avoided intellectually disabled individual are considered a benefit, then the lost lifetime contribution of the potential individual lost in the miscarriage should be considered as a cost. It is obvious that a complete cost–benefit calculation is impossible. And, even if it were, the problem is far from solved. If, for example, the costs to society for caring for a certain group is shown to be more expensive than a prevention programme, *exactly how much more expensive* would it have to be to justify prevention? At least in the earlier analyses the hidden premise seemed to be that prevention is justified if it can be shown to save money, however small the difference.

Thirdly, a new feature in a recent large summary of antenatal screening for Down syndrome was that formal comparisons of the cost of screening and the cost of lifetime care were not made at all, even though otherwise extensive data on the cost-effectiveness of the screening were provided (Wald *et al.* 1997). The justification was, in the words of the report: ' . . . because the reason for screening is not to save the costs of care. The purpose is to give couples the opportunity to avoid having a child with severe abnormality, not to make financial savings to the health services' (Wald et al. 1997, p. 226). This statement brings us back to the tension between the public health model and the reproductive autonomy model, which was discussed in the chapter on prenatal diagnosis. The researchers seem to have abandoned economic justification for prevention overtly, but this attitude does not resolve the issue completely, since the logical connection between screening and the incidence of the particular condition remains.

Societal burdens that are not quantifiable in monetary terms are more abstract and seem to escape quantification in general and comparability in particular. This discrepancy brings us to the so-called incommensurability problem. I shall return to it shortly after presenting examples of the non-economic adverse social effects of a genetic screening programme.

Examples of adverse social effects

Sickle-cell anaemia is inherited as a recessive trait, and it has a highly variable clinical expression, from full life with minor symptoms to painful crises, organ damage and early death. The prevalence of the gene is high among black populations.

Several states in the USA implemented mandatory screening programmes for sickle-cell disease in the early 1970s. The programmes were even considered an attempt at genocide against the black population. Irrespective of the validity of the claim, they were said to divide the black community over the desirability of testing (Whitten 1973).

The programmes also raised concern due to the great influence they had on screening-positive carriers, many of whom were discriminated against for purposes of marriage, employment and insurance (Boss 1993). Carriers also often experienced their status inappropriately, being told that they had a mild form of sickle-cell anaemia, when, in fact, carrier status implies difficulties only in some special circumstances like hypoxia under anaesthesia or flying at high altitudes in unpressurised aircraft (Behrman and Vaughan 1987).

Still other problems occurred with the programmes. They included inaccurate diagnoses by some physicians, when individuals with the trait were told only that they 'had' sickle-cell anaemia. Some medical institutions performed the test routinely, without prior consent, and the programmes were often established without a counselling component. As Whitten (1973, p. 318) has remarked, simply determining and informing a person of the possession of the sickling gene is potentially worse than not testing at all.

Incommensurability

At first sight, it would seem obvious that a plurality of moral values implies the impossibility of solving ethical dilemmas. Moral commensurability has, however, been the aim of many thinkers both in the utilitarian and Kantian traditions. Recent virtue theorists (e.g. Nussbaum) have argued for the vanity of this quest and have, in general, criticised the tendency of modern moral philosophy to concentrate on the general features of human life, thus ignoring the particular aspects of the human situation (Hallamaa 1994).

The meaning of the term incommensurability needs some clarification. In *Well-being* (1986) James Griffin discusses incommensurability and distinguishes several forms of it.

In a *strong* sense of the word it could mean that two items cannot be compared quantitatively at all (i.e. they cannot fit onto any scale of measurement). In a *weaker* sense it could mean that no amount of one sort of item can equal, in some respect of quantity, a certain amount of another. In addition, when we speak about the incommensurability of values, we should clarify what we mean by 'values' in this context. If our understanding of 'value' is very broad, incommensurability between values is inevitable.

The strongest sort of incommensurability is incomparability, where two values are so far from each other that they seem unrankable. We do not, however, argues Griffin (1986), find values that are *strictly* incomparable. We should not exaggerate the difficulty in ranking values. We can and do compare, for example, pain and accomplishment, although they cannot be measured on the same scale and the comparison may be difficult. If the pain is great and the accomplishment minor or vice versa, we have an easy choice. A human life has no equivalent, but keeping the speed limits where they are inevitably leads to deaths on the roads.

The next strongest form of incommensurability allows a comparison of values, but there is one trumping value that outranks the others. Could autonomy or liberty serve as such a trumping value? No, since most of us would sacrifice some liberty or some autonomy to avoid great pain or some other kind of catastrophe in our lives.

A weaker form of incommensurability would seem to follow from the problem of weighing values. When we think that it takes a great deal of happiness to outrank a fairly small amount of misery, we seem to use two distinct scales. But, argues Griffin (1986), neither of these scales is the ultimately important one. *Behind* them is a single scale, on which prudential values are ranked, and the special weighing disappears.

Thus incomparability and trumping are too strong, and weighing is a distraction. Is there any form of incommensurability for Griffin? Yes, there is, but not so that some *types* of values outrank other types. But we do, for example, rank a certain amount of life at a very high level above any amount of life at a very low level. This attitude leads to the general formulation of incommensurability: enough of A outranks any amount of B.

How is all this relevant for the societal burden argument? If we believe in Griffin's (1986) argument, we should not, without careful scrutiny, accept statements about the impossibility to compare the burden an intellectually disabled child brings to society and the burden of trying to prevent that disability.

There are, of course, easy cases in which the former greatly outweighs the latter. Preventing ID due to congenital hypothyreosis costs money and causes short-term anxiety to parents whose child tests falsely positive. After an adequate explanation these parents easily accept this minor psychological harm as a price for the possibility to catch the true positives in due time.

Much harder are the cases in which the burden of accepting intellectually disabled children and the burden of screening and terminating them prenatally must be compared. In a society which accepts abortion for *some* reason, a comparison has already been made. We cannot claim incommensurability between these burdens unless we deny the moral possibility of abortion totally.

Commensurable or not, the non-economic burdens at the societal level are rather abstract and not as easily definable as at the level of the family. However, there is no doubt that such burdens exist and they should be considered.

Beyond quantification have been said to be such potential consequences of screening as possible conflicts between a pro-screening majority and a minority of women or families who refuse testing (Kass 1985). Obviously they would be difficult to quantify, but would such a conflict be incommensurable in the preceding sense? We can imagine other analogous situations in which the interests of a majority and a minority clash: if a minority group thinks that it is against its ideology or religion to pay taxes, the majority overrules its belief. Here we see the difficulty of claiming the superiority of a *general* value like autonomy. In the taxation example *economic* autonomy is obviously commensurable, and there are limits to it. However, in the screening example, reproductive autonomy is incommensurable in the preceding sense. At least in our present Western societies no amount of societal advantage would outrank the reproductive autonomy of women to say no to prenatal screening. There are, of course, more subtle pressures, but overt coercion is out of the question.

If social worth is considered a sufficient criterion for establishing a prenatal screening programme for conditions leading to ID, it is also justified to ask why the issues should not be broadened and discuss the infanticide of the newborns whose diagnoses were missed prenatally. Or why it should not be broadened further and apply the social worth criteria later in life and consider active euthanasia for these individuals? The latter questions are important, but I shall leave them for the moment and return to them in Chapter 8 on the moral status of foetuses and the intellectually disabled.

I have now considered various aspects of the societal burden argument and conclude that it alone has thus not proved to be strong enough to justify the prevention of ID. Cost–benefit calculations may never be accurate enough to form a basis for prevention, and, even if they did, there remain important social values that should be considered.

Quality of life of persons with intellectual disability

One way to formulate the quality of life argument goes like this: individuals with ID often have a low quality of life. Especially those who have associated physical handicaps may have an extremely low quality of life, in some cases even to the extent that life can be considered worse than death. These kinds of lives are not worth living; therefore preventing states leading to such lives is justified.

There are several questions involved here. Firstly, what do we understand by quality of life? As usual, there is no agreement among philosophers and social scientists about the criteria for a good quality of life. Secondly, can quality of life be adequately assessed? And if it can, what is the best way to do it for the intellectually disabled? Thirdly, does the quality of life argument provide general justification for the prevention of ID?

What is quality of life?

The term 'quality of life' was originally introduced in the 1950s to criticise policies aiming at unlimited economic growth (Musschenga 1997). The critics saw that material values only could not suffice in making people's lives satisfactory. A decade later the term proved useful in the medical context, when it became necessary to find measures for success that were not quantitative. In the field of social science the rival term 'well-being' has been widely used, but in medicine and health care 'quality of life' became the term of choice (Musschenga 1997). In fact, the end of the twentieth century has witnessed a quality of life movement with whole textbooks and a speciality journal dedicated to the subject (McLaughlin and Bjornson 1998).

With reference to ID, issues of quality of life have been raised in two contexts. Firstly, in the context of prevention, usually in the form of selective abortion. Quality of life has also been cited as justification for withholding medical treatment from infants with severe disabilities and even for euthanasia. Secondly, quality of life has been discussed and researched in the context of the lives of intellectually disabled persons (e.g. when changes have occurred in their living or working conditions).

Traditionally, quality of life has been considered an entity that can be measured in terms of *objective* or *subjective* indicators. Among the first, social indicators such as nutrition, air quality, incidence of disease, crime rates, health care, educational services, divorce rates and the like can be used. The second possibility is to define quality of life as a subjective measure of perceived satisfaction. In fact, several articles in the AAMR book on quality of life (Schalock and Siperstein 1996) stress the nature of quality of life as a subjective experience. It may or may not be something that people *think* about, and generally thoughts are devoted to quality of life mostly during 'the highs and lows of life' (Taylor and Bogdan 1996, p. 16).

The distinction between 'objective' and 'subjective' is not, however, entirely unambiguous, and it resembles the philosophical distinction between 'needs' and 'wants', which is not a settled issue (Allardt 1993). Subjective indicators of quality of life tell about people's wants. Objective indicators, however, may refer to both needs and wants. In empirical social science the distinction between objective and subjective standpoints is a concrete dilemma. When, for example, housing standards are measured, one could rely on objective measures like the space available or one could ask the respondents whether they are satisfied with their housing conditions (Allardt 1993).

The nature of quality of life as an *entity* has also been questioned. Schalock (1996) has suggested that it should be seen more as a process or flow or an organising concept. Taylor and Bogdan (1996) borrow the distinction between the *sensitising* and *definitive* concepts suggested by the sociologist Blumer. The latter refers precisely to what is common in a class of objects, while the former lacks the specification of attributes. Quality of life would be a sensitising concept, and a qualitative approach to research would be preferable to a quantitative approach.

Some sceptical voices in the ID field have questioned the whole concept of quality of life on various grounds. The origin of the concept is rooted in the concern to encapsulate the well-being of populations rather than that of individuals. The use of the term has also become charged, thus inhibiting rational debate. Some writers have even cautioned against the use of the quality of life term altogether (Luckasson 1990, cited by Borthwick-Duffy 1996, p. 108, Hatton 1998).

The term 'quality of life' may be rather recent, but the issue is not. The concept of happiness is not equal to quality of life, but the present discourse on the latter has its roots in the earlier discourse on the former. Classical utilitarianism was interested in the maximisation of happiness, roughly the same as subjective quality of life, and, for it, how happiness was distributed in society was irrelevant. Present-day utilitarianism is a 'complex cluster of moral theories based on the principle of maximising welfare' (Gillon 1994, p. 22) and a general discussion on utilitarianism is beyond this book. In Gillon's words: 'simplistic criticisms based on simplistic accounts of the theory are inappropriate' (Gillon 1994).

The quality of life issue can be approached from other perspectives than strictly utilitarian ones. According to Amartya Sen, essential is not what people have but what they do with what they have. Thus he has suggested the 'capability approach', which is concerned with people's actual abilities to achieve various valuable functionings as a part of living (Sen 1993). 'Functionings' represent parts of the state of a person – in particular the various things that he or she manages to do or be in leading a life. Sen has also presented the idea of a pluralistic approach to a good life in which each component could be thought of as an independent vector. These components may be broadly comparable between individuals (objective measures) even though the resulting aggregate understanding of the goodness of a person's life is highly individual and subjective (Coulter 1997).

Sen's approach has much in common with the empirical work done on the quality of life in social sciences. Relevant for our purposes may be the *basic needs* approach categorised by the catchwords Having, Loving and Being. This approach combines both subjective and objective aspects of well-being and has been generally developed in Scandinavia, especially by the Finnish sociologist Erik Allardt.

Having refers to the material conditions necessary for survival and for avoiding misery (Allardt 1993). It covers such needs as nutrition, air, water, protection against diseases and the like. Empirically, it is measured by indicators denoting economic resources, housing and working conditions, health and education.

Loving stands for the need to relate to other people and to form social identities. The level of need satisfaction in this area is assessed by measures denoting attachments to family and the local community, relationships with workmates, active patterns of friendship and the like.

Being stands for the need to integrate into society and to live in harmony with nature. Personal growth and alienation represent the positive and negative aspects of Being, respectively. Empirical indicators measure, for example, the extent a person can participate in decisions and activities influencing his or her life, opportunities for leisure-time activities, meaningful work and so forth.

Allardt's Having–Loving–Being distinction resembles in turn the conceptual framework developed in the ID context (Hughes and Hwang 1996). Although the researchers found 44 different definitions of quality of life, they were able to identify 15 dimensions that were present in most of the definitions. In the same book, researchers from Wales aggregated these dimensions into a model of three dimensions: objective life conditions, subjective feelings of well-being and personal values and aspirations (Felce and Perry 1996). They ended up with the following definition (p. 68):

Quality of life is defined as an overall general well-being that comprises objective descriptors and subjective evaluations of physical, material, social, and emotional well-being together with the extent of development and activity, all weighted by a personal set of values.

These dimensions interact with each other and are potentially interdependent. Thus, for example, a change in a person's values may initiate changes in satisfaction and precipitate changes in objective circumstances.

The definition of quality of life cannot be separated from the purpose that the definition is needed for. The objective descriptors may obtain more weight if the purpose of the study is to compare a group of intellectually disabled persons with another group of non-intellectually disabled persons. On the other hand, subjective evaluations will be crucial, if the life of a person or a group in place X is compared with later life in place Y. As with the AAMR definition of mental retardation, this one is also too wide to define exact categories. Thus it might perhaps be best regarded as a framework that allows several applications depending on the particular purpose of the use of the term.

Assessing quality of life

Before going to the actual measurement or assessment of quality of life, I shall consider shortly the purpose of this activity. At least three different purposes can be identified (Häyry 1990).

Firstly, the purpose may be related to the fair allocation of scarce health resources. In situations in which not all those in need can be treated, medical personnel should choose to treat the patients who benefit most, in terms of both the quantity and the quality of their remaining lives. The unit of comparison can be a patient, a treatment, a physician, a hospital, an illness, a branch of medicine and the like. An inherent ethical problem with this motivation for the measurement of the quality of life is its ageist, as well as racist and sexist, nature. The young could easily be preferred to the old, and, since race, sex and social status are determinants of health, these factors could also be employed in allocation decisions. The 'quality of life' concept in the context of resource allocation seems to serve mainly as a camouflage for purely economic decision-making (Häyry 1990).

Secondly, the purpose of the measurement may be to facilitate clinical decision-making. A typical example would be a consideration of whether a particular medical procedure would produce better quality of life for an individual. The introduction of quality to quantity considerations has, of course, been a progressive move in the assessment of various therapies, but QALYs (quality-adjusted life-years) are also accompanied by obvious problems. If various forms of treatment for an individual patient are compared, the main ethical issue is *who* determines the quality in question.

Thirdly, the assessment of quality of life may be associated with assisting patients towards autonomous decision-making concerning their own lives. The issue of autonomy is an obvious problem in the context of ID, and in most cases proxies or care givers assist in the assessment.

From the preceding discussion, it should be obvious that there cannot be a single indicator of the quality of life of a person. The objective descriptors are relatively easy to measure and can, in most cases, be quantified and thus compared. Assessing the subjective aspect of quality of life is far more problematic, and the association between life conditions and subjective well-being can be weak. The following problems occur if only subjective quality of life is assessed (Felce and Perry 1996).

Firstly, reports of subjective well-being may be more a reflection of a person's internal temperament than of external conditions. Significant changes in life conditions may induce only temporary changes in reports of well-being.

Secondly, satisfaction is a measure of comparison. A slave who is satisfied with obtaining some freedom is still a slave. Empirical research has shown that residents from a range of living environments, which differed markedly as to objective characteristics, expressed equally high satisfaction with their circumstances. This finding shows the importance of including both subjective and objective standards in the assessment of quality of life.

Cultural factors should also be considered when the quality of life of an individual or a group is assessed. The role of values may differ significantly from culture to culture and, for example, the concept of loneliness may be interpreted and experienced quite differently in individualistic and collectivist cultures (Keith 1996).

The effect of culture has been shown in empirical research. For example, the quality of life scores of Tongans living in the USA more nearly resembled those of people with ID than those of American adults without retardation (Keith 1996). There is an obvious parallel here to the measurement of IQ. Ignoring cultural factors creates a bias that easily results in systematically lower scores among test subjects who come from a culture different from the one the test has been developed for.

ID brings about some specific methodological issues in the measurement of quality of life. The principal problem in comparisons with non-intellectually disabled people is the difficulty to determine the individual's perspective and values (Coulter 1997). Acquiescence, a strong tendency to say 'yes' to most questions, and a low consistency of answers to multiple-choice questions are two examples of such measurement problems. The significance of the former has been, however, questioned in some recent research (Matikka and Vesala 1997).

There are alternative solutions to the methodological problems. Identifying optimally effective questioning techniques, correcting statistically for response bias, using proxies and, in general, using multiple methodologies increase the validity and reliability of the assessment (Heal and Sigelman 1996).

A different approach to the assessment of quality of life has also been developed to overcome the shortcomings of cross-sectional studies or longitudinal studies with only two or three points of measurement. The ethnographic approach aims at a relatively continuous measurement in which the researchers attempt to comprehend and interpret the phenomena under study as faithfully as possible (Edgerton 1996). The researchers have prolonged contact with the people in question and become, if only relatively so, a natural part of their lives. This kind of methodology has, for example, shown that younger people with intellectual disability who are new to life in community settings are unhappy much of the time. On the other hand, these same people become happier as they grow older and their lives stabilise. In addition, ethnographic studies suggest that a subjective sense of well-being may derive more from personal attributes than from the impact of the environment (Edgerton 1996).

Quality of life and intellectual disability

What, then, is the position of the quality of life argument?

The issue is far more complicated than the formulation of the quality of life argument would suggest. Saying that 'individuals with ID often have a low quality of life' does not mean much unless several details are clarified.

Firstly, what is understood by ID here? Does the claim refer to anybody who scores below −2 SD on a standardised IQ test or to anybody who meets the criteria of the AAMR definition (see Chapter 2)? In both cases it is obvious that the group is too heterogeneous for such generalisations. If we look at the definition given earlier for quality of life, no reason can be found as to why ID per se would decrease the quality of life of the individual. The very mildly intellectually disabled or so-called borderline cases may be the only ones who suffer from their inferior intelligence, not being able to manage in the open work market and feeling rejected by their peers. On the other hand, they do not feel that they belong to the world of the intellectually disabled. The suffering these persons experience reflects the attitudes of the environment to a great degree and does not originate from low intelligence as such. It is easy to imagine, for example, a rural community in which such a person could find his or her place and would not suffer any more than the others. We can also imagine some suffering at the other extreme of the IQ distribution: a highly intelligent child or youngster might as well suffer from rejection by peers.

Secondly, what exactly is meant by quality of life and how has it been measured? Does the claim refer to objective or subjective standards, have cultural and value issues been taken into account and so forth? If objective standards have been used, what are they, and, if the intellectually disabled have been found to score lower than the non-intellectually disabled, what is the link between disability and low scoring? The possible causality should also be questioned if subjective standards have been used: do those who are unhappy feel bad because they are intellectually disabled or because they have been poorly cared for (Rose-Ackerman 1982)? In addition, it can be questioned whether burdens *external* to the individual should be counted in calculating one's quality of life at all (Boss 1993). These burdens can be considerable in the form of a lack of socio-economic or familial support to establish a minimally satisfactory life. Counting these external burdens would, however, lead to problematic conclusions, since it would then be logical to consider selective abortion in cases in which the prospect of the foetus without a diagnosed condition leading to disability would be miserable due to unfavourable social conditions.

Thirdly, claims about low quality of life with the intellectually disabled should include an explanation about the comparison group. Low when compared to whom? Low at point t in time or low for a lifetime? Research literature on quality of life of the intellectually disabled population is abundant, but the object of the studies has seldom been to compare the intellectually disabled population with a non-intellectually disabled population. Instead, the studies often evaluate quality of life in changing living conditions or in relation to particular procedures. I have come across only one paper in which the quality of life of the intellectually disabled was compared with that of the general population (Matikka 2000). After acknowledging the methodological difficulties, the author concluded that, in general, the intellectually disabled are as satisfied with their lives as the rest of the population. The former did, however, experience physical violence and stress more often than the latter.

Fourthly, if research shows a lower score for an intellectually disabled population, what is the magnitude of the difference and what is the relevance of the magnitude? In the afore-mentioned American study the mean scores for non-Tongans without retardation, Tongans without retardation and non-Tongans with retardation were, respectively, 99.8, 90.6 and 90.9. The differences were certainly statistically significant if the sample size was not very small, but it is worth asking how relevant the difference was, for example, from the point of view of prevention.

The second part of the quality of life argument referred to those who also have physical handicaps and stated that they may have an extremely low quality of life, in some cases even to the extent that life can be considered worse than death.

ID is often accompanied by physical handicaps, which may cause considerable suffering. The suggested justification for selective abortion in these cases refers to survivability or the possibility of a pain-free existence. The former issue poses the problem of the length of 'normal' life that is considered worthwhile. Is it 6 months, as in Tay–Sachs disease, or 40 years, as in Huntington's disease? Or should we perhaps consider the ratio of 'normal' to 'abnormal' years? And, in the end, there always remains the question of whether the individual actually suffers in such a way that it would overcome the desire to continue life.

When trying to imagine what an intellectually disabled person feels, we may too easily think what *we* would feel if we suddenly developed similar mental and physical characteristics. This, of course, does not tell anything about the feelings of the actual person, who, in most cases, has had the qualities for a lifetime.

In addition to the aforementioned reservations concerning quality of life and its measurement, there is another fundamental issue that I have already briefly mentioned, namely, the question of whether the concept should be used at all in the context of ID.

In a recent article this question was approached seriously, although the author acknowledged the obvious shortcomings of abandoning the concept altogether

(Hatton 1998). He presented two critiques of the 'emerging quality of life consensus' with which he obviously refers mainly to recent work within the AAMR, which is largely presented in the two volumes already mentioned (Schalock *et al.* 1996, 1997).

According to the first critique insuperable problems arise when one attempts to assess subjective quality of life. The first of these problems is the disenfranchisement of people with severe intellectual disability. If one has little or no communication skills, it is hardly possible to assess the genuinely subjective quality of life. The second problem arises from the meanings different participants bring to quality of life assessments. There is evidence suggesting that people with ID may regard quality of life interviews as a test of their fitness to remain in their community-based houses rather than as research interviews about their life that will have no potentially negative consequences (Hatton 1998). The third problem relates to the aforementioned question of the stability of subjective quality of life. If subjective well-being is largely influenced by personality, major long-term alterations dependent upon improvements in objective life circumstances are not to be expected (Hatton 1998).

According to the second critique the quality of life approach, which generally claims to liberate people from a medical model, may paradoxically serve to *extend* professional control over the lives of people with ID (Hatton 1998). The history of services for people with ID can usually be characterised by significant improvements in the form of de-institutionalisation and integration. There is an alternative interpretation, however, which claims that changes in service provision reflect, at least in part, battles for professional dominance rather than advances that liberate people. The change may have brought an *increased* professional grip over their lives. Abandoning the quality of life approach, as well as many other forms of measurement and assessment applied to people with ID, would, according to this critique, lead to benefit for these people. For example, the rights to privacy, dignity and control over one's own life would be increased.

Although abandoning difficult concepts like quality of life (or ID altogether) may sound attractive, it also creates obvious problems. If we accept historical relativism and consider progressive development only as a sign of change in the balance of professional dominance, then the attempts to do anything progressive lose their meaning (Hatton 1998). Practical consequences may also result from this kind of view. The intellectually disabled will no longer be labelled, but they may become invisible and disempowered in many important contexts, like economics, politics, welfare and health (Hatton 1998).

Abandoning issues of quality may also lead to a one-sided enhancement of issues of quantity. How important both are is reflected in an article and a related editorial in the *American Journal of Public Health* in 1996. The article reported a study in which the predictors of mortality among severely disabled children with ID were assessed. Own home residence and community care facilities were associated with a 25% increase in mortality when compared with institutions (Strauss *et al.* 1996). The accompanying editorial discussed possible methodological flaws and stressed the lack of outcomes other than mortality (Durkin 1996). As the editorial notes, 'no advocate for children or for public health in general would recommend institutionalisation as a strategy for reducing mortality in children without mental deficiencies' (Durkin 1996, p. 1360). Quality of life may be difficult to measure and hard to compare, but it is perhaps an even more important outcome than pure mortality. And last, but not least, it may in fact be impossible or extremely difficult to avoid totally the notion of quality of life. We might try to do so but still implicitly refer to it (Hoedemaekers 1998).

The quality of life argument is commonly referred to in discussions about selective abortion and the prevention of ID in general. As we have seen, the content of the term 'quality of life' has often not been specified and even the whole concept has been criticised as questionable. The argument is often used loosely, without details about the measurement or comparison in question being specified. Obviously, it is not meaningful to refer to the quality of life of the whole intellectually disabled population, as it is questionable to refer to *any* particular characteristic of that population which even escapes exact definition. Measuring and comparing quality of life may be meaningful with reference to small subgroups with relatively similar mental and physical characteristics. Even then one should carefully consider the causal origin of the associations found. Stanley Hauerwas (1986, pp. 171–2) may have been right when he wrote: 'Perhaps what we assume is not that the retarded suffer from being retarded but rather, because they are retarded, they will suffer from being in a world like ours.'

Concluding remarks

We have seen that very different arguments have been presented to support the prevention of ID. Some of them focus on the individual, some on the family and some on society. Some arguments consider suffering, some economic good. In the medical context they are often presented superficially, ignoring the complexity of some more-or-less hidden assumptions behind each argument. I shall now briefly consider the strengths and weaknesses of each of the arguments in justification of prevention at the level of an individual or society.

The greatest weakness of the eugenic argument is the vagueness of terms like 'eugenic', 'genetically normal' and 'genetic health'. Since there is apparently no standard human genome to be defined by science, drawing the demarcation line between 'normal' and 'abnormal' will always be a value judgement. The argument also seems to assume an unproblematic notion of what is the common good. There is an obvious utilitarian rationale according to which greater good will be achieved automatically if humankind is able to rid itself of certain faulty genes. In the final analysis the question is very much about the balance between the good of the individual and the good of society. Both can be measured in terms of many different indicators (e.g. economic, health-related or autonomy-related), the weighing of which results in different policies.

The problem with the foetal-wastage argument lies in its assumptions about nature and natural. As we have seen, nature is not consistent in selecting which embryos or foetuses have good prospects for life. Nature does not necessarily eliminate genes leading to ID, as the example of the reproductive success of women with fragile X syndrome shows. In addition, the supporters of the foetal-wastage argument have failed to demonstrate why natural should be considered good in general or with respect to spontaneous abortions in particular. The goals of medicine are manifold and the achievement of these goals may entail enhancing, restoring or acting against natural processes.

The family burden argument may be more successful than the two previous ones, if two conditions are met. Firstly, familial reproductive autonomy is given high value, and, secondly, a psychological or economical burden is accepted as a justification for abortion. However, we should separate two issues, the *general* justification for the prevention of ID (e.g. in the form of introducing nationwide programmes) and justification in *particular* cases. In the former case, the argument is weaker because there is substantial variation in the psychological and economic burdens and especially the economic burden is highly determined by the nature of the health and social services available in a particular society. In the latter case, if obvious burden can be anticipated in a particular family, the argument is strong. If a society accepts abortion on request, there are no convincing arguments to deny it from parents willing to influence some qualitative features of their offspring. This statement does not, however, mean that health care providers should have a duty to perform prenatal diagnosis on any kind of request. The other side of respecting parental autonomy is supporting parents' right to give birth to children who will be intellectually or physically handicapped. The replaceability argument, according to which parents would in some cases have a duty to abort a foetus with a condition known to lead to ID, was shown to be weak because it ignores the particular contexts of real life, where decisions are made.

The societal burden argument was shown to be problematic for several reasons. Cost–benefit calculations, which have been overtly or covertly used to justify prevention programmes may perhaps never be accurate enough to form a basis for prevention. The recent means of justifying screening, not in terms of cost-effectiveness but instead in terms of the enhancement of reproductive autonomy, does not abolish the economic issue, since it is highly improbable that a cost-*in*effective screening programme would be established *only* to enhance autonomy.

Non-economic societal burdens are more difficult to measure, but they are real and do not necessarily escape commensurability totally. Even a value like autonomy can be commensurable in the sense that some amount of autonomy may be considered worth sacrificing if enough of something good is gained. However, no amount of societal good, at least in present Western societies, can be considered enough to outrank the specific autonomy of pregnant women to say no to prenatal screening or testing.

Finally, the quality of life argument was also shown to be problematic in many ways. The concept of quality of life is far from clear and has been used in many meanings referring to subjective or objective aspects of an individual's life or sometimes a combination of these. Despite these difficulties much research has been done in this respect and something can be said about the quality of life of intellectually disabled persons.

Firstly, it has not been shown that the intellectually disabled in general would have a considerably lower quality of life than the rest of the population. In fact, the existing empirical evidence points out that the differences are minor. Secondly, it may be that it is not meaningful to refer to the quality of life of the *whole* intellectually disabled population. Thirdly, even if a subgroup or an individual can be shown to have a markedly low quality of life, we must be careful with conclusions about causality, since the low quality may not be a necessary consequence of ID but of environmental origin.

8

Moral status and intellectual disability

What is moral status?

The concept of moral status is used widely, yet there are no clear-cut definitions for it. People, animals, things, ideas and the like are referred to as having moral status. It may be low or high and it can be compared (i.e. there are various *degrees* of moral status). Moral status can also be thought of as *intrinsic* or *conferred*.

The vagueness of the concept of moral status is obvious when one looks at the following examples:

- X has moral status → It is always wrong to destroy X.
- X has moral status → It is prima facie wrong to destroy X.
- X has moral status → X has a right to respect (life, help, care, etc.).
- X has moral status → Y has a moral obligation with regard to X.

Although moral status seems to escape an exact definition, it is plausible that people in general think along the following lines. If something has moral status it is worthy of moral consideration (Edwards 1997), and we have, or can have, moral obligations towards it (Warren 1997).

The concept of moral status can be thought of as 'a means of specifying those entities towards which we believe ourselves to have moral obligations, as well as something of what we take those obligations to be' (Warren 1997, p. 9). The concept is *general* by nature. We usually ascribe moral status to *members* of a group, not merely to specific individuals (Warren 1997).

A wide consensus seems to prevail about the moral status of many things and beings. On one hand, stones and other inanimate objects are usually considered to have no moral status at all (Warren 1997); on the other hand, adult human beings with normal intelligence are considered to have full moral status. This consensus has not been or is not, however, complete.

Firstly, in some philosophical schools, the idea of moral status or its generality is rejected. Moral nihilism denies the possibility of moral principles. According to ethical egoism each moral agent has obligations only toward itself, and moral subjectivism sees claims about moral matters as a matter of individual opinion (Warren 1997).

Secondly, there are examples of cultures and philosophies in which some inanimate things like stones are considered sacred, which is obviously a form of moral status (Warren 1997).

Thirdly, not all adult human beings with normal intelligence have been or are given full moral status. Until the twentieth century women were given lower moral status than men by most great names related to the history of Western philosophy. In our time race or sexual orientation are examples of traits used to deny full moral status.

I have so far deliberately used the example of 'adult human beings with normal intelligence' and thus not mentioned the main topic of this chapter, namely, the relationship between intelligence and moral status. As we have already seen in Chapter 4, attitudes towards ID have varied from neglect to respect. Intelligence has been and is used as a criterion for full moral status. Thus, in addition to racism and sexism, there is something that might be called *intelligism* (Vehmas 1999a). This chapter focuses on the question of whether this intelligism can be morally justified.

Criteria for moral status

The moral status of a being or a thing can be based on its *intrinsic* or *relational* properties. Philosophical theories about moral status can refer to a single property or to several properties as a basis for moral status. Mary Ann Warren (1997) calls the former uni-criterial theories, and she suggests a multi-criterial account for moral status. I find her criticisms about the uni-criterial theories plausible and will review them briefly, concentrating, however, on theories with special relevance to the main topic of my book.

Intrinsic properties that have been proposed as single criteria for moral status are life, sentience and personhood. They all look attractive in presenting a relatively clear and simple criterion for moral status. A closer look reveals, however, problems with each.

Life

Life as the only criterion for moral status leads to serious problems. Firstly, it is not obvious what should be counted as a living thing and is thus worthy of moral respect (Warren 1997). Secondly, if we wish to continue living at all, it is not, in practice, possible for us to give equal moral status to all living things. Each time we brush our teeth, for example, we obviously destroy millions of living organisms.

While having life does not seem to work as the *only* criterion for moral status, it could work better as *one* of the criteria for moral status. If having life guarantees some moral status, then *any* destruction of life – however primitive – would require some justification. Below I present the multi-criterial account for moral status, and having life will be one of these criteria. But first let us go to the important issues of sentience and personhood.

Sentience

According to *Webster's Comprehensive Dictionary* one meaning of sentience is 'capacity for sensation or sense perception'. In the philosophical context, however, the word is used in a somewhat narrower sense, referring to 'capacity to suffer or experience enjoyment or happiness' (Singer 1993, p. 58).

For the philosopher Peter Singer, the limit of sentience is 'the only defensible boundary of concern for the interest of others' (Singer 1993, p. 58). Furthermore, 'If a being is not capable of suffering, or of experiencing enjoyment or happiness, there is nothing to be taken into account' (Singer 1993, p. 57–8).

I shall leave aside the discussions about animal consciousness and their general capability to feel pain. For me, it is simply plausible, for example, from the evolutionary point of view, that at least so-called higher animals can feel pain in a way that is equivalent to or greatly resembles the human experience.

Strictly speaking, we cannot be sure which animals are sentient. In the same way, of course, *I* cannot be sure whether any other human being is sentient or whether my car is or is not sentient. There is, however, evidence that supports the claim that a particular entity is sentient in the preceding sense (Warren 1997). Having a nervous system and sense organs indicative of perceptual ability, responding to noxious stimuli in certain ways (crying, howling, moaning, escaping, etc.) and the presence of neurochemicals that, in humans, are related to experiences of pain and pleasure are examples of such evidence. For the purpose of my book, it is not important where we draw the line between sentient and non-sentient animals, but the preceding evidence suggests that at least mammals and birds are sentient (Warren 1997).

According to Singer (1993), the principle of equal consideration of interests is a basic moral principle. And 'an interest is an interest, whoever's interest it may be' (Singer 1993, p. 21). The importance of one's interests does not depend on his or her abilities or other characteristics apart from the characteristic of having interests. Sentience is the only relevant factor here; for example, sex, race or species are not. Non-sentient organisms may have needs, but they do not feel pain or pleasure and cannot 'mind' what happens to them (Warren 1997).

There is a special group among sentient beings, the members of which are self-aware and capable of reason – *persons*. The lives of persons are more valuable to themselves than the lives of other sentient beings to themselves. Thus killing a sentient being is wrong, but killing a person is more seriously wrong than killing a non-personal sentient being (Singer 1993).

This very brief description of Singer's views cannot, of course, do justice to his work, which has been developed over decades and presented in several books and articles. I hope, however, to have presented the main idea in such a way that its problems can be understood in the light of the criticism that follows.

At least three kinds of problems arise from sentience as the *only* criterion for moral status. Firstly, the view ignores the benefits of ascribing moral status to non-sentient living things and plant or animal species. Even from a strictly utilitarian point of view this stance may lead to greater happiness for a greater number of sentient beings.

Secondly, and more important from the point of view of my book, Singer seems to consider the moral status of beings in relative isolation, as if their relationships with the world outside would be almost irrelevant. Singer, as well as some other utilitarian bioethicists (e.g. Harris), emphasise that emotions should not have an essential role in our moral judgements. This view has been challenged in feminist ethics and the ethics of care (Warren 1997). Our moral obligations cannot be understood in isolation from our human intuitions and feelings (Noddings 1984). An obvious example is the care of parents for their children. In Noddings' words, 'A philosophical position that has difficulty distinguishing between our obligations to human infants and, say, pigs is in some difficulty straight off. It violates our most deeply cherished feelings about human goodness' (Noddings 1984, p. 87).

Thirdly, equal consideration of the interests of all sentient beings precludes activities essential to human health and survival (Warren 1997). This preclusion is obvious at least in the case of small invertebrate animals, most of which are 'neither cute nor cuddly'. They are seriously harmed through ordinary domestic and agricultural activities, and even acting as a peaceful gatherer of wild plant foods would require sometimes putting human interests ahead of those of other sentient beings (Warren 1997).

Personhood

The concept of person has been very central in bioethical discourse during the past three decades. The history of the concept is long, 'starting in Roman antiquity, maturing in the Christian Middle Ages and consolidating in Modern Times' (Welie 1998, p. 210).

Originally the Latin term *persona* referred to the mask used in Roman theatre. In later Roman times it began to denote the particularity of individuals. According to Welie, it was Boethius who presented the first formal definition of personhood: 'the person is the individual substance of a rational nature' (Boethius cited by Welie

1998, p. 212). Later, in the Middle Ages, the term began to refer also to dignity and legal duties.

No single exact definition of 'person' exists in modern bioethical discourse. In any case, being a person carries a strong conceptual link to having full moral status (Warren 1997). Being 'alive' or 'sentient' is at least to some degree a *scientific* question, but whether one is a person is not a scientific but a philosophical question.

In our everyday speech we use the term 'person' rather loosely and with different meanings. For example, we do not usually refer to animals as persons. On the other hand, people who, strictly taken, do not yet or no longer have the capacity for moral agency are referred to as persons in our everyday speech (Warren 1997).

In philosophy, however, the terms 'person' and 'personhood' have been given specific meanings, depending on the context and frame of reference of the writer in question. Martyn Evans has claimed that, in philosophical and public debate, unfamiliar interpretations of ordinary concepts (like 'person') may 'gain an influence which they do not deserve – partly because of the mystique and authority which is attracted by any idea that sounds technical' (Evans 1996, p. 24). This technical term is then used as though it could settle moral issues in an objective, pseudo-scientific way. Evans also presents a collection of recent definitions of 'person' or 'personhood' and summarises their essential features as follows:

1 'The person' as a value-free description (at least, initially).
2 Personhood as a sign of being valuable.
3 Personhood as the chance of *feeling* valuable.
4 Personhood as cognitive capacity.
5 Personhood as cognitive and affective capacity.
6 Personhood as moral wholeness.
7 Personhood as possession of neurological structures.
8 Personhood as really useful, or, as the benefit of the doubt.
9 Personhood as the ground of conscious identity.
10 Personhood as individual humanity.
11 Personhood as the possibility of consciousness.
12 Personhood as conscious mental life.
13 Personhood as metaphysical, first and foremost.

The list clearly demonstrates the wide variety of meanings these concepts have had in contemporary philosophy. It also helps us to see that the question 'What is a person?' is not empirical but is instead conceptual (Evans 1996).

These conceptual issues do not arise in a vacuum but do so because of a need for a definition that can be applied to a particular problem (Evans 1996). Evans argues further that at the root of the conceptual disagreement (of the definition of 'person') is a moral disagreement about how in fact different individuals ought to be treated.

Jaana Hallamaa ended up with very similar conclusions in her thesis *The Prisms of Moral Personhood*. 'Person' is not a theoretically 'innocent' concept. It 'includes an implicit normative aspect in the sense that it states what is morally important and relevant and what can be left to one side... Person as a moral term implies our central normative commitments, it does not offer a neutral ground for solving moral disagreements' (Hallamaa 1994, p. 257).

It was probably Michael Tooley who introduced the radically new definition of the concept of person that has been used by several utilitarian thinkers (Tooley 1972). For Tooley the concept of a person is 'a purely moral concept, free of all descriptive content' (Tooley 1972, p. 40). To be a person means the same as to have a serious moral right to life. An organism possesses a serious right to life only if it possesses the concept of a self as a continuing subject of experiences and other mental states and it believes that it is itself such a continuing entity. It follows that foetuses, newborns and severely intellectually disabled or demented humans are not persons in this sense but that adult individuals of some higher species of primates are. Obviously the most problematic conclusion would be that, in a conflict situation, we should prefer the life of an adult chimpanzee to the life of a newborn human being. I strongly doubt whether Michael Tooley would be willing to go this far in practice.

Different strategies have been used to avoid this difficulty. Engelhardt, for example, introduced the concept of a *social person*. These individuals, because of their capacity to interact in social roles, are accorded some of the rights of persons strictly (Engelhardt 1986). Thus personhood is no longer the sole criterion for moral status; instead, other criteria referring to the world outside are introduced as well.

Apparently, then, the most serious problem in using personhood as the only criterion for moral status is the same as the aforementioned second problem related to the concept of sentience. Judgements about moral status are made in isolation, as if the world outside and the relationships between the individual in question and his or her environment would be irrelevant.

This can be seen as an example of the problems of an individualistic philosophy in bioethics in general and an individualistic approach to ID in particular.

Jos Welie has written an extensive critique of the libertarian approach to bioethics, which, according to him, 'implies the denial of the significance of fellowship for the theory of ethics. It overestimates the freedom and manipulative powerfulness of humans while underestimating the positiveness of intersubjective care' (Welie 1998, p. 194). Welie does not write about the intellectually disabled in particular, but his general criticism about the trumping status of autonomy in modern bioethics has obvious implications for their status, too. Welie himself turns to continental philosophers like Levinas, Heidegger and Marcel in building up a new foundation for clinical ethics.

Steven Edwards has argued that the low moral status often accorded to people with ID derives from individualism (Edwards 1997). He identifies two main components in the individualistic position: the ontological view concerning the nature of the self and the normative view concerning the nature of a moral agent.

According to the ontological component of individualism, 'the existence of the self and the identity of the self does not depend upon the existence of anything else beyond the self' (Edwards 1997, p. 34). An obvious classic of this kind of thinking is Descartes, but Edwards mentions also John Rawls as a contemporary example of ontological individualism. The normative component of individualism states that the ideal moral agent is fully autonomous, thus being able to make his or her own decisions about a good life.

Both of these aspects of individualism refer to *independence* in their own ways. The self is an independent entity if its existence does not depend on the existence of other selves (Edwards 1997). One is *socially* independent if one does not need the concern and care of others. This has obvious implications for the status of the disabled, who, if any, are in many ways dependent on other people in their daily lives.

The issue of dependence can, however, be seen in a totally different light. Instead of the disabled being considered a marginal group, they can be seen as *distinctively human* because of their dependence on other people (Vehmas 1999*b*). Earlier, I referred to Jos Welie's book, in which he discussed the issue more generally. The particular chapter in which he brings in Heidegger and Marcel is titled 'Solitarity or Solidarity?', which captures nicely the essence of the philosophical dispute. Steven Edwards, in his turn, seeks the answer in the philosophy of Charles Taylor, whose view of self is radically at odds with the individualist view (Edwards 1997).

Relationships and moral status

Being alive, sentient or a person are *intrinsic* properties of individuals (i.e. it is logically possible to have them without reference to the existence of other beings). Moral status has also been based on *relational* properties like an entity's social and ecological relationships or the relationship of caring (Warren 1997).

According to some representatives of environmental ethics, all our moral obligations arise from the fact that we are members of communities, biological or social (Warren 1997). One possible line of argument claims that the autonomy of a short-lived individual should not be preferred to the dynamic life form of its species, genetically persisting over millions of years (Honderich 1995). The so-called deep ecologists want to preserve the integrity of the biosphere for its own sake, irrespective of the possible benefits for humans (Singer 1993). The emphasis is not on living organisms but is instead on entities like species, ecological systems or the whole biosphere. Furthermore, the deep ecologists think that the value we place on our own lives should be placed on the life of every living thing.

Again, this kind of thinking adds some important aspect to our moral understanding, but it is problematic to justify basing the moral status of entities *solely* on, for example, the role of the species of these entities within a social or biotic community. Firstly, as Singer remarked, we have a strong intuition that 'the rights to "live and blossom" of normal adult humans ought to be preferred over those of yeasts, and the rights of gorillas over those of grasses' (Singer 1993, p. 282). Secondly, the relationship between the moral status of a species and individual representatives of that species is not clear. Thirdly, neither is it clear where the border is between entities that can or cannot be regarded as 'holistic'. An atom could well be considered a holistic system if we were in the size class of quarks. On the other hand, in the size class of the Milky Way, the holistic system would probably be the whole Universe.

Another line of argument that refers to relationships as a basis for human morality can be found in the feminist ethics of caring (Noddings 1984). According to it, the traditional approach to ethics that begins with a discussion of moral principles, judgement and reasoning is not the best starting point. Instead, moral status is seen as a function of *caring*, a fundamental emotional relationship that is feminine by origin. Reason sets priorities and helps us to determine the ways to meet the needs of those we care for; the motivation to care is, however primarily emotional, not rational. We are 'at the centre of concentric circles of caring. In the inner, intimate circle, we care because we love' (Noddings 1984, p. 46). When we move outward in the circles, we encounter first those for whom we have personal regard; further on are those we have not yet encountered.

Noddings illustrated the femininity of this approach by citing some examples from the literature, one of which is the story of Abraham and his son Isaac at the Moriah Mountain. According to her, a woman could not have written this Biblical account, where God asks Abraham to sacrifice Isaac. A mother would not have acted as Abraham did, nor would a Mother-as-God have demanded what this Father-God did.

The caring ethics sees us *related* at the very heart of our being: 'My very individuality is defined in a set of relations. This is my basic reality' (Noddings 1984, p. 51). We are free to reject the impulse to care, but it may not lead to happy consequences. We are not naturally alone but are instead in a relation or in relations from which we derive nourishment and courage.

Noddings' theory contains important elements that should be considered when the moral status of a being is evaluated. It does not, however, work alone. At least the following problem arises: if moral obligations depend on the individual's possession of specific empathic capacities, what about the persons who lack such capacities completely? Do they have moral obligations at all, and, if they do, how can these obligations be justified? If moral rules and principles are totally rejected, we are lost in cases in which empathy does not guide us (Warren 1997).

A multi-criterial approach to moral status

All the earlier-mentioned uni-criterial theories contain important insights, but they do not provide necessary *and* sufficient conditions (i.e. an adequate definition of moral status). In the following discussion, I present a brief description of a multi-criterial account of moral status by Mary Ann Warren (1997). I find it a plausible and powerful tool with which to examine the moral status of various beings and entities. I present the seven principles of moral status with only short comments on each. In the rest of this chapter I apply this account to various groups of human beings, in particular foetuses, newborns, children and adults, with potential or actual ID.

1 The Respect for Life principle: Living organisms are not to be killed or otherwise harmed, without good reasons that do not violate principles 2–7

This principle gives at least some moral status to all living things. However, beings that have a stronger moral status than can be based upon mere organic life do no wrong if they harm, for example, some micro-organisms while taking care of themselves or preparing food or the like. Later principles specify factors that define what counts as a sufficiently good reason for harming a living thing.

2 The Anti-Cruelty principle: Sentient beings are not to be killed or subjected to pain or suffering, unless there is no other feasible way of furthering goals that are (1) consistent with principles 3–7; and (2) important to human beings, or other entities that have a stronger moral status that can be based on sentience alone

Death is a greater harm to sentient beings than to non-sentient beings. 'Pain is pain, no matter who feels it' (Bonnie Steinbock, cited by Warren 1997, p. 153). The principle does not require us to treat all sentient beings as our moral equals, but it demands a stronger justification for harming organisms that are sentient than what is required in the case of non-sentient organisms. It is likely that sentience is a matter of degree. The intensity of the experience of pain probably does not differ, but beings that are subjects of their lives have more to lose than mentally less sophisticated beings.

3 The Agent's Rights principle: Moral agents have full and equal basic moral rights, including the rights to life and liberty

This principle probably has long-term value for humans although applying the principle may not always maximise happiness. Language is a prerequisite for moral agency, because moral concepts and principles require it. Most human beings are therefore obvious moral agents, but some higher primates may be such, too. On the other hand, newborns or profoundly intellectually disabled persons who do not have language are not moral agents in this sense.

4 The Human Rights principle: Within the limits of their own capacities and of principle 3, human beings who are capable of sentience but not of moral agency have the same moral rights as do moral agents

Principle 3 does not imply that only moral agents have basic moral rights. Principle 4 gives these rights to human beings that are not yet, will never be nor are any longer moral agents. Human beings become moral agents only through a long period of dependence upon human beings who are already moral agents. 'Persons essentially are second persons, who grow up with other persons' (Annette Baier, cited by Warren 1997, p. 164). Therefore, it is impractical to deny full moral status to, for example, newborns. It is, of course, also emotionally offensive to most people. The issues of infanticide and the moral status of the intellectually disabled are dealt with later in this chapter.

5 The Ecological principle: Living things that are not moral agents, but that are important to the ecosystems of which they are part, have, within the limits of principles 1–4, a stronger moral status than could be based upon their intrinsic properties alone; ecologically important entities that are not themselves alive, such as species and habitats, may also legitimately be accorded a stronger moral status than their intrinsic properties would indicate

According to this principle some plants and animals have a stronger moral status than their intrinsic properties would suggest, because their species is ecologically important and endangered by human activities. The principle also allows more than instrumental value for, for example, earth, air, water and biological species.

6 The Interspecific principle: Within the limits of principles 1–5, non-human members of mixed social communities have a stronger moral status than could be based on their intrinsic properties alone

We usually feel that we have stronger moral obligations to animals we have established social relationships with. Although they are not fully moral agents, they resemble such in their behaviour. They may, for example, show affection, loyalty, courage and patience. Something that resembles a promise is made when a relationship between a human being and, for example, a dog is established.

7 The Transitivity of Respect principle: Within the limits of principles 1–6, and to the extent that is feasible and morally permissible, moral agents should respect one another's attributions of moral status

This principle allows some moral status for entities that would not have such according to principles 1–6. A graveyard is an example of such an entity.

Moral status before birth

Although the development in genetics has been astonishing during the past several years, no therapeutic breakthroughs have taken place. A great number of conditions leading to more- or less-severe ID can be diagnosed prenatally, but almost always the options are either to abort the foetus or accept the condition in one's offspring. If induced abortion is totally banned on moral grounds, the prevention of these conditions is ruled out. If, on the other hand, a human being is thought to gain moral status only when capable of valuing his or her own life, there are no moral problems with preventing such conditions. These extremes are not subscribed to by many, since their practical implications are hard to accept and there are also theoretical problems involved with both positions.

These problems arise from trying to solve the moral problems of abortion by referring to some criteria the foetus either meets or fails to meet. There are, however, relevant *relational* properties, especially the dependence on the body of a sentient moral agent. The moral status of this agent is also at stake and so may be the position of the entire human species. Applying the multi-criteria approach may help to clarify the issue.

Embryos and young foetuses

I used the terms 'embryo' and 'foetus' a few times in the previous chapters without defining them. In general, an 'embryo' refers to the first stages of development after fertilisation; in the human species it usually refers to the first 2 months. Thereafter it is called a 'foetus'. This terminology is, of course, a matter of convention, and sometimes the terms pre-embryo and embryo proper are also used. By a 'young foetus' I mean a foetus until about 26 weeks of gestation. The reason for the use of this term is empirical and will be explained later.

Embryos and young foetuses have some moral status according to the Respect for Life principle. They are not, however, moral agents and cannot have the status the Agent's Rights principle would allow. Embryos are not sentient and the Anti-Cruelty principle cannot be applied to them. The possible sentience of foetuses needs more scrutiny.

Obviously we cannot *know* for sure whether a foetus is sentient (i.e. able to suffer or experience enjoyment or happiness). Much is, however, known about some of its physiological reactions and at least something can be inferred from that information.

Firstly, young foetuses lack the necessary structures to feel pain. First sensory experiences are not possible until the thalamocortical tracts have developed (26th gestational week). Evoked potentials are not possible until the 29th gestational week, and therefore we can only speculate about possible pain between weeks 26 and 29 (Vanhatalo 1999).

Secondly, the activity of the frontal cortex is needed for the cognitive dimension of pain. The area is activated during the first year of life. Therefore, the pain we feel may not be equal to the pain a newborn feels (Vanhatalo 1999).

Thirdly, the foetus, however, reacts to painful stimuli much earlier. The first reactions to somatic stimuli appear at 7.5 gestational weeks. These reactions can be strong and non-specific, and they can be similar to reactions to non-painful stimuli (Vanhatalo 1999).

Fourthly, hormonal, metabolic and autonomic responses to painful stimuli can be controlled with analgesics. Such control has been shown in premature babies in surgery or intensive care (Vanhatalo 1999).

All this information implies that foetal pain may not be the only relevant factor here. It seems obvious that foetuses are not sentient before 26 weeks, but even before that some sensory stimuli may be harmful to the development of the foetus. If it is aborted, it cannot be said to have suffered, but, if it continues life, it can have been harmed.

So far we have discussed the principles referring to the *intrinsic* properties of the foetus. They are not, however, the only relevant principles here. The Transitivity of Respect principle states that moral agents should respect one another's attributions of moral status to the extent that is feasible and morally permissible. Since some people regard foetuses as having full moral status, respect for these people gives at least some moral status to foetuses and embryos. However, this moral status is limited by the moral rights of women according to the Agent's Rights principle (Warren 1997).

Does it matter what the foetus looks like? The answer is partially yes, on the following grounds. A young embryo does not look human, in fact it resembles animal embryos, like worms, tadpoles or pigs (Richardson and Reiss 1999). Only later does it begin to look more human. When foetuses reach the limit of viability, they look very much human. This does not bring sentience or moral agency to them, but it does raise strong feelings in most people. Seeing one's offspring in the screen of an ultrasound machine is a strong experience. Again, according to the Transitivity of Respect principle these more-human-looking foetuses should have a higher moral status than the less-human-looking ones. This principle also explains the common view that the moral status of the foetus becomes *gradually* stronger. But, at least until they are sentient, their moral status is lower than that of their mothers, due to the Agent's Rights principle.

Does it matter whether the embryo or the young foetus is a future person with ID? Such embryos and foetuses do not differ essentially in their morphological characteristics from those with potentially normal intellectual development. In their genetic characteristics these two groups differ: one group carries a potential for normal, the other for more or less compromised intellectual development.

They should, however, have *some* moral status according to the Respect for Life principle. Although some people think that the moral status of intellectually disabled persons is lower than that of non-disabled persons, the Transitivity of Respect principle does not work in that direction. I take it for granted that moral agents' respect for 'one another's attributions of moral status to the extent that is feasible and morally permissible' refers to *positive* moral status. The principle does not mean that the moral status of an entity would be a bit lower with every person willing to give it such a low status.

Older foetuses

If the afore-cited scientific reasoning about the prerequisites for sentience is correct, the foetus becomes sentient at about 26 gestational weeks. Thus it reaches an important milestone in moral status, and the Anti-Cruelty principle should be applied: it should not be killed or subjected to pain or suffering, unless there is no other feasible way of furthering goals that are (1) consistent with principles 3–7 and (2) important to human beings, or other entities, that have a stronger moral status than could be based on sentience alone. The Human Rights principle should also be applied: within the limits of their own capacities and of the limits of principle 3, human beings who are capable of sentience but not of moral agency have the same moral rights as do moral agents.

Obviously it is the mother of the foetus who, in most cases, is the person with stronger moral status and whose interests may be at stake. It is not perfectly clear what the 'limits of their own capacities' mean in the Human Rights principle, but at least being situated inside an agent with full moral rights limits the capacities of the foetus. Although the moral status of the foetus has become stronger with advancing age, it is not equal to that of its mother. If it were, decisions would be difficult in situations in which carrying on a pregnancy seriously risks the life of the mother.

There is a grey area in gestational age during which the foetus is probably viable outside its mother, but (if the preceding scientific reasoning is correct) not sentient. The lower limit of viability is currently at about 24 weeks, although there are a few exceptions at 23 or even 22 weeks (of course, the estimates of gestational age are not exact). What should we think about such foetuses?

Viability has been an important milestone with reference to foetal rights. For example, in the famous *Roe* v. *Wade* decision, the United States' Supreme Court established viability as the point after which states may prohibit abortions that are not deemed necessary to protect the life or health of the woman (Warren 1997).

The concept of viability is somewhat ambiguous. Sometimes it refers to a point in time when the foetus may survive outside the womb *without* any special neonatal intensive care. On the other hand, it may refer to a possibility to survive *with* the help of such intensive care (Warren 1997). This ambiguity is not, however, decisive.

Although it is true that the great majority of the now surviving babies born before 26 weeks would die without special care, there have been occasional cases in which they have survived even before today's technology was available.

There are several reasons why the foetuses in this grey area (viable but not yet sentient) should have a rather strong moral status, at least to the point that abortion is prohibited without obvious threat to the mother. Firstly, the moral status of the foetus has become gradually stronger with advancing age, for example, its appearance being very human. Secondly, viability would introduce obvious moral problems into the abortion procedure itself. There would be three options: kill the foetus inside the womb, kill it outside the womb or do nothing except take it out. The first two would violate strongly the ethics of the medical profession, which, according to the Transitivity of Respect principle, should be considered here. The third option would result in a few foetuses surviving after all – very probably with severe handicaps if not taken to intensive care. Of course, aborting viable foetuses, taking them to intensive care and, if they survive, giving them up for adoption would be an option, but then one could seriously ask why not give the foetus a few more weeks for a better chance to survive without handicaps.

Moral status after birth

Birth does not make a difference with respect to moral agency. The newborn baby is no more a moral agent than the foetus inside its mother's womb. Both are to be respected according to the Respect for Life principle, the Anti-Cruelty principle and the Human Rights principle. The Transitivity of Respect principle also adds something to the moral status of both groups.

Birth does, however, make a crucial difference when the interests of the foetus or newborn and the interests of the mother are compared. Protecting the interests of the individual *before* birth always compromises the interests of the mother; after birth the two individuals are physically separated and such compromising does not take place.

Also, a newborn baby immediately acquires a social role that differs from the role of the foetus just a few minutes earlier. Thus, while the intrinsic properties relevant to moral status do not change at birth, there are highly relevant changes in some relational properties.

The concept of ID can not be applied to newborns or young infants. However, these children sometimes have conditions that lead to ID later in childhood. This development can often be predicted with high probability, but even in these cases the degree of disability remains uncertain.

There are no obvious factors that would make the moral status of these children lower than that of children with no known condition probably leading to ID. The issue of infanticide has, however, been raised in this context.

Newborns and young infants

Newborn babies are surely not persons in the sense that Michael Tooley defined personhood. According to him, they do not have a serious right to life because they lack an essential feature, namely, 'the concept of a self as a continuing subject of experiences and other mental states', neither do they believe that they are themselves such continuing entities (Tooley 1972, p. 44). Tooley does not discuss the relevance of ID to moral status, but it does come up, for example, in the work of Peter Singer and Helga Kuhse, who more or less directly stress the relevance of intelligence to moral status (Kuhse and Singer 1985, Singer 1993). The issue of active and passive euthanasia is one of the central topics in both books, but I shall concentrate only on the discussion concerning intelligence and its relevance to moral status.

Kuhse and Singer (1985) describe the case of Brian West, who was born in 1980 with Down syndrome and oesophageal atresia (i.e. no connection between the back of the mouth and the stomach). He was operated on soon after his first birthday, but without the consent of his parents. Still, oral feeding could not be attempted until he was almost 2 years old. It was never very successful, and Brian died of brain damage due to severe breathing problems in December 1982. During his short life Brian spent a lot of time in hospital and in intensive care, had several operations and obviously suffered a lot. Afterwards it is easy to think that his life would probably have been better if it had been short and without the operations. The outcome, of course, was not obvious at the time of the decision to operate.

There are many burning ethical issues here, and it is especially tragic that there was no consensus about treatment choices between Brian's parents and the doctors in charge. What is important for my issue here is the reasoning of Kuhse and Singer about the relevance of Down syndrome to treatment decisions.

According to them it was relevant in two ways. Firstly, physical characteristics related to Down syndrome, like poor muscle tone and increased susceptibility to infections of the upper respiratory tract, were probably associated with the outcome. The former may have complicated swallowing in the newly reconstructed oesophagus, and the latter may have contributed to Brian's additional complications after surgery. Brian's father also suggested that the reduced intellectual capacities of a child with Down syndrome may have compromised his learning to eat after surgery.

Secondly, Kuhse and Singer wrote:

But, quite apart from these medical factors, Down syndrome is surely relevant to the decision to operate because it means a reduced potential for a life with the unique features which are commonly and reasonably regarded as giving special value to human lives … It might be justifiable to run some risk of the kind of misery Brian experienced, if there were a fair chance of a reasonably normal life; the same risk might not be justifiable if the best that could be hoped for was the reduced potential of the life of someone with Down syndrome. (Kuhse and Singer 1985, p. 143)

These words indicate that (future) ID as such means lower moral status to Kuhse and Singer. Letting such a child die is more justifiable than letting a child with (future) normal intelligence die. And, to take one step further, because there is no crucial difference between killing and letting die, killing a (future) intellectually disabled infant is more justifiable than killing a child with (future) normal intelligence.

While one can hardly question the misery of the life of Brian West, there are other points where Kuhse and Singer's views are questionable. Firstly, the assumption that the quality of life related to ID per se must be lower than the quality of life with normal intelligence is clearly wrong. I am not aware of empirical research comparing the quality of life of people with Down syndrome to that of other intellectually disabled individuals or people with normal intelligence. However, the commonly held view that Down syndrome is associated with a joyful and positive character may well be true. In fact, if it is true, a utilitarian should *prefer* the life of an individual with Down syndrome to the life of someone without this syndrome.

Secondly, the reasoning of Kuhse and Singer seems to imply that the value of life decreases gradually with decreasing intelligence. What would then be the lower limit of intelligence that would guarantee full moral status? What about the individual with subnormal intelligence but not ID (according to current definitions)? What about extremely intelligent individuals and their quality of life?

Thirdly, the context in which one is born and lives is very important for one's happiness. Simo Vehmas (1999*b*, p. 115) has presented the following clarifying example (for which he acknowledged John Lizza):

Suppose A is a boy without intellectual disabilities who grows up in an impoverished environment with bad familial and social relationships, whereas B has Down syndrome but grows up in an excellent environment with good social and familial support. Which one has the prospects for a more satisfactory life? Probably the child with Down syndrome, especially if the other child grew up in a neighbourhood where statistics showed that a high percentage of the young males end up in prison or dead. Would Kuhse, Singer and Rachels think it permissible to kill infants born in impoverished environments because the prospects for their lives would be much worse than for those born in a more affluent environment?

How does this all look in light of the multi-criteria approach to moral status? We have seen that foetuses can gain moral value from sources other than their intrinsic capacities only. In addition, birth is a significant milestone, after which the moral status is even stronger. The newborn or a young infant gains moral status from many sources. The Respect of Life principle, the Anti-Cruelty principle, the Human Rights principle and the Transitivity of Respect principle all guarantee the moral status of these people although they cannot yet be claimed to be moral agents and have rights according to the Agent's Rights principle. ID is not relevant here. Of course, the individual may have a physical condition that makes life miserable, and it can be seriously asked whether palliative and basic care with a short life is better than intensive and operative care with a (possibly) longer life. However, even though ID would be associated with this particular condition, it is the physical condition, not the intellectual capacity, that is the major determinant of the quality of life of the individual.

Children and adults with intellectual disability

The concept of ID is not meaningful for young infants, neither can they be called moral agents. During late infancy or early childhood the individual gains moral agency, and it also becomes possible to test his or her intelligence. We have seen that possible future ID is not relevant to the moral status of a foetus, newborn or young infant. How is the situation for older children and adults with *actual* ID? Does the degree of disability affect the moral status of an individual?

Steven Edwards has introduced the concept of the Low Moral Status (LMS) claim, according to which human individuals with intellectual disabilities are accorded, justly or unjustly, a moral status that is lower than that accorded to intellectually able human individuals (Edwards 1997, p. 31). He presents four considerations as evidence in support of this claim.

Firstly, future ID is usually considered to justify the termination of pregnancy. This does not necessarily imply, as Edwards notes, that the moral status of children and adults with ID is therefore compromised. It may, however, be so that, in practice, the treatment of foetuses with features associated with disabilities reflects the general attitude towards children and adults with such features. John Harris wrote in 1985 about this dilemma as follows:

Most people would not, I suppose, think that mentally or physically handicapped individuals are somehow less valuable than others, and yet anyone who thinks that the detection of handicap in the foetus is a good reason for abortion, must accept that such an individual is, or will become, less valuable than one without such handicap, less valuable because less worth saving or less entitled to life. (Harris 1985, p. 7)

Harris returned to this issue more deeply in 1998 and, interestingly, he seems to have changed his views. As we saw in Chapter 5, he argues against a *necessary* connection between prenatal screening and the quality of life of disabled persons (Harris 1998b). Accepting the abortion of foetuses with certain conditions does not necessarily imply that lower moral status should be accorded to born individuals with such conditions. Although I agree with Harris here, it is still worth noting that, in *practice*, there may well be an association between attitudes towards these two groups.

Secondly, until recently, it was an accepted practice to let, for example, children with Down syndrome and associated gut malformations die instead of performing life-saving operations. In the USA the so-called Baby Doe regulations clarified the situation and condemned such practice. English law remained ambiguous on this subject until 1990 (Edwards 1997).

Thirdly, the notions of personhood popular among utilitarian philosophers (see the earlier discussion) may be thought of as supporting the lower status of individuals with ID. However, even if the extreme views on personhood were adopted, there would be implications only for the status of the profoundly intellectually disabled, who are a small minority of the population with ID. I shall consider their position in more detail later.

Fourthly, the terminology applied may carry implicit messages concerning moral status. Edwards mentions terms like 'mentally subnormal', 'mentally retarded' and 'mentally deficient'. The message of these terms is not, however, so obvious. The choice of term may reflect political correctness in a particular context rather than moral connotations.

The LMS claim, as presented by Edwards, describes the moral status *accorded* to individuals belonging to this group of people, rather than to their *actual* moral status (i.e. the moral status which an individual may be thought to possess independently of the moral status accorded to him or her). I shall now consider the actual moral status of these people in the light of Warren's multi-criteria approach.

It is obvious that the great majority of people with ID are moral agents, also persons in the sense of, for example, Tooley (possesses the concept of a self as a continuing subject of experiences and other mental states and believes that it is itself such a continuing entity (Tooley 1972, p. 62)). Therefore, the Agent's Rights principle should be applied to them, and their basic moral rights should not differ from those with normal intelligence.

It was mentioned earlier that language is a prerequisite for moral agency, because moral concepts and principles require it. This may be so, but there is no clear-cut demarcation line between individuals who possess language and those who do not. There are many examples of severely physically disabled individuals who have been thought to be profoundly intellectually disabled too, but whose cognitive abilities have turned out to be normal when adequate means of communication have become possible. Christy Brown, the author of *My Left Foot*, is the most famous example.

Although the classification is difficult, there are individual human beings who are not and will never become moral agents. The Human Rights principle should be applied to them: 'within the limits of their own capacities and of principle 3 (the Agent's Rights principle) . . . they have the same moral rights as do moral agents'. Conflicts of interest similar to those between a foetus and its mother cannot take place here. However, situations can be thought of in which we have to choose between the rights of a human moral agent and a profoundly intellectually disabled human being. In such a case the rights of the former would weigh more, since the agent would have a stronger moral status due to the Agent's Rights principle.

Furthermore, a hypothetical case could also be thought of in which the rights of a non-human moral agent and a severely intellectually disabled individual would be in conflict. I am not referring to E.T. or a future super-computer but to intelligent higher primates. Analogously with the preceding case, the rights of the moral agent should be preferred. However, the supporters of the non-human individual would bear the burden of proof of showing that the intellectually disabled individual definitively lacks the characteristics of a moral agent.

Concluding remarks

The concept of moral status is useful and often referred to, although mostly indirectly or implicitly. We cannot escape comparing the moral value of entities and beings, although it sometimes creates difficult dilemmas.

In philosophical theory various properties have been proposed to form the basis for moral status. If a single criterion is used, the view easily becomes too narrow. I have found Warren's recent multi-criterial account for moral status plausible and useful both in general and with reference to ID in particular.

Embryos and young foetuses gain some moral status from the Respect for Life principle. The present or future life situation of the mother (or the family) may, however, sometimes justify the killing of the foetus, because the moral status of the mother is stronger than that of the foetus. Possible future ID does not make any difference here.

Older foetuses that have reached sentience have higher moral status, since the Anti-Cruelty principle should be applied to them. Again, future ID does not make a difference here. In the few weeks' grey area, when the foetus is viable but not yet sentient it should have a rather strong moral status, at least to the point that abortion is prohibited without obvious threat to the mother.

The newborn or a young infant gains moral status from another principle. The Human Rights principle guarantees them a higher moral status than foetuses can have. Still, ID is only a future possibility in this group and does not make a difference with respect to moral status.

It is only in the group of children and adults with actual ID in which very low intelligence may be relevant to one's moral status. While the great majority of intellectually disabled persons can be said to be moral agents in the full sense of the term, some individuals with profound ID obviously lack the qualities necessary for moral agency. The Human Rights principle should be applied to them, but in a possible conflict situation the moral status of a full moral agent would be stronger.

9

The ethics of prevention in practice: three syndromes

Down syndrome

Down syndrome (DS) was first described as a separate entity in 1866 in an article titled 'Some observations on an ethnic classification of idiots' by British physician John Langdon Down (Booth 1985). He had observed that a large number of congenital idiots resembled Mongols and therefore he described them as Mongolian idiots.

Although the syndrome has carried Dr Down's name ever since, he was not, however, the first to associate intellectual disability and Mongolian racial characteristics. Already in 1844 Robert Chambers had suggested a theory of degeneration, according to which the human brain goes through various stages of development from animal forms to 'Negro, Malay, American, and Mongolian nations and finally is Caucasian' (Chambers R. *The Vestiges of the Natural History of Creation* (1844), cited by Booth 1985, p. 4). Chambers suggested that 'parents too nearly related tend to produce offspring of the Mongolian type – that is, persons who in maturity still are a kind of children' (Booth 1985).

The 'official' history of DS is thus a little more than 150 years old. It is not clear whether the syndrome had been recognised earlier, since histories of childbirth and midwifery omitted children born with physical impairments (Booth 1985). Almost certainly the syndrome existed, however, long before its recognition.

John Langdon Down not only described the physical characteristics of this group of people, but also drew attention to the features of their personality:

They have considerable powers of imitation, even bordering on being mimics. They are humorous, and a lively sense of the ridiculous often colours their mimicry. They are usually able to speak; the speech is thick and indistinct, but may be improved greatly by a well-directed scheme of tongue gymnastics. (Down 1866, cited in Carr 1995, p. 1)

The view that there was a connection between DS and the Mongolian race was challenged by several researchers at the turn of the century, but influential writers were still revising and elaborating Chambers' ideas about human development, in which the Mongoloid stage precedes Caucasian adulthood, in the 1930s.

Direct observation of human chromosomes became possible in the 1950s, and in 1959 Lejeune first described a chromosomal abnormality for individuals with the syndrome. He noted that they had an extra chromosome 21, the total number being 47 instead of 46 chromosomes, and the syndrome became known also as trisomy 21.

The process that leads to trisomy originates during meiosis (a phase in cell division), when non-disjunction takes place and trisomic cells result. Non-disjunction may take place during mitosis (another phase in cell division) and result in mosaicism (i.e. the presence of more than one population of cells with different chromosome numbers in the same individual). Most (95%) individuals with DS have 'regular' trisomy 21, and approximately 1% are mosaic, the remainder being the result of translocation, in which two chromosomes have joined together (the extra chromosome 21 has joined to, for example, chromosome 14) or an exchange of chromosomal segments between two different chromosomes has taken place (Kingston 1994).

The incidence of disjunction is known to correlate with maternal age, but the reason for this correlation is unknown. It is thought to be due to some aspect of the ageing oocyte, although it may occur at any age.

Characteristics

DS is characterised by typical facial features, short stature and intellectual disability. Congenital anomalies are present in several organ systems. For example, congenital heart disease is diagnosed in approximately 40% of the children, and malformations of the gastrointestinal tract in 12% (Pueschel 1990). Surgical treatment is possible in a great majority of the cases.

The childhood years of an individual with DS may be complicated by infections, increased susceptibility to leukaemia and disorders of the thyroid glands. The high risk of leukaemia continues through life, but DS also means a decreased risk of solid tumours in all age groups (Hasle *et al.* 2000).

In adolescence most individuals enjoy good health. In Carr's follow-up study at ages 11 and 21 the severity of illnesses was more pronounced in the DS group but the number of children who had suffered serious illnesses was comparable between the DS group and the control group (Carr 1995). However, significantly more children in the control group had suffered a serious accident. The overall conclusion of Carr was that the differences between the groups were not as striking as expected. This statement referred to both subjective estimates of health (as 'general health' reported by the mother) and objective measures such as hospital appointments or medication.

Conceptions of intellectual capacity in DS have varied from time to time, and from the beginning of the twentieth century both pessimistic and optimistic views have been expressed. A common assumption has been that all are severely intellectually disabled (IQ under 50), but this opinion is far from the truth. On the basis of several studies it has been estimated that the chance for an IQ figure above 50 is 30–55% (Booth 1985). People with DS differ from one another to an extent similar to that seen in a non-disabled population (Carr 1995).

The popular view sees people with DS as cheerful, friendly, affectionate and fond of music. There are methodological problems in addressing this issue, for example, the question of how far this kind of stereotype is self-fulfilling. Carr (1995) has summarised some recent studies according to which children with DS are seen as more affectionate, outgoing and more positive in mood but also as less persistent and distractible than non-disabled children.

The life expectancy for a baby born with DS has increased considerably. In 1929 it was 9 years and in 1947 it was still only 12 years. At that time only a few lived to be mature adults (Carr 1995). Today the situation is different. A Canadian report estimated in 1988 that about 44% and 14% of liveborn infants with DS will survive to 60 and 68 years, respectively (Baird and Sadovnick 1988). When compared with survival in the general population, the survival in this group is poorest during the first year of life. Thereafter, a plateau appears in the survival curve until the age of 44 years, after which survival falls more quickly than among the general population (Baird and Sodovnick 1988). A few individuals survive, however, for a very long time, the oldest being reported to be 86 years of age (Carr 1995, p. 4).

There is no specific therapy for DS, and to my knowledge no breakthroughs are to be expected in the foreseeable future. Some research is, however, in progress. A small open trial on four adults with DS was conducted in the USA to test the effect of donepezil, a cholinergic agent, on cognitive performance. The rationale behind the trial was the neuropathological and neurochemical similarities between DS and Alzheimer's disease and the effect of the drug on symptoms of the latter. The results of the trial were modest but the authors suggested that a larger placebo-controlled trial with cholinergic therapy was needed for persons with DS (Kishnani *et al.* 1999).

Epidemiology

As has already been noted, the probability of having a baby with DS correlates with maternal age. Various figures have been presented from different parts of the world, but everywhere the general trend of increasing prevalence with advancing maternal age can be found.

Table 9.1 shows the birth prevalence of DS in various age groups and the percentages of all births and DS births occurring in each group in England and Wales

Table 9.1. Maternal age and Down syndrome (DS) (England and Wales 1979–1985)*

Maternal age (years)	Prevalence of DS births per 1000 pregnancies	Percentage of all births in this group	Percentage of DS in this group
Under 20	0.4	9	5
20–24	0.4	30	17
25–29	0.5	34	25
30–34	1.0	19	27
35–39	2.2	6	18
40–44	5.1	1	7
45 or over	8.1	0.1	1
all ages	0.7	100	100

*Adapted from Rose (1992).

Table 9.2. Results of prenatal screening for Down syndrome (DS) in Maine between 1980 and 1993*

Variable	1980–1985	1986–1990	1991–1993
Cases of DS expected	97	95	60
Cases of DS identified			
By amniocentesis alone			
No. of cases	9	20	10
No. of cases terminated	8	19	10
By serum screening			
No. of cases	0	15	30
No. of cases terminated	0	10	27
After birth – no. of cases	78	71	30
Reduction in prevalence of DS among live births (%)	7	23	46

*Adapted from Palomaki and Haddow (1996).

(Rose 1992). It also demonstrates the fact that most children with DS are born to women under 35 years of age.

The effect of prenatal diagnosis on the birth prevalence of DS was small in the early days of prenatal diagnosis, when it was based on maternal age only. The introduction of serum screening has changed the situation in many areas, as Table 9.2 shows. The influence of screening on the birth prevalence of DS is, of course, dependent on the detection rate and the percentage of women willing to have the test. Still, it depends on the abortion rate among women who have tested positive. The latter has been around 90% in several studies.

The highest reported detection rate has so far been 93.7% with a false positive rate of 5% (Sheldon 1999, Bahado-Singh *et al.* 2002). It can be expected that the tests will become more sensitive and more specific, and, if the uptake of the test does not decrease considerably, the effect of screening for the birth prevalence of DS will be larger than earlier. However, the number of individuals with DS will not decrease for decades because of the increase in life expectancy that has occurred during the past few decades.

Development of prenatal diagnosis

The first prenatal diagnosis of DS was made in the late 1960s, and the practice to offer the possibility for amniocentesis or chorionic villus biopsy for women 35 years of age or older was disseminated widely in the developed world during the following two decades. As early as 1973, it was proposed that complete prevention of the syndrome could be achieved by screening every pregnancy by amniocentesis (Carr 1995). Due to the obvious technical and, especially, ethical problems of such a programme, such complete screening has thus far not taken place anywhere.

Screening according to maternal age turned out, however, to be ineffective, since the majority of children with DS were and are born to younger women, simply because they bear so many more children than older women. In 1987 it was reported that a low serum alpha-fetoprotein concentration of the mothers is a marker of risk for DS (Copel and Bahado-Singh 1999). Thereafter rapid progress has been made in the field, and several other serum markers have been introduced. The most commonly used markers are alpha-fetoprotein, human chorionic gonadotropin and unconjugated estriol. Second-trimester ultrasonography can also be used to identify affected foetuses. Many different protocols are in use, and in 1998 France was the only country to have a national screening programme for DS (Cuckle 1998).

As has been noted earlier in the chapter on prenatal diagnosis and screening, the ethical issues involved are far more complex than in screening for, for example, cancer, the gains and costs being hard to compare.

The economic cost of DS screening consists of ultrasonography, biochemical tests, consequent invasive tests, and the working time of obstetricians, midwives, general practitioners and genetic counsellors. The classical gain in the cost–benefit analyses has been the amount of money saved in the lifetime costs of caring for people with DS. It has recently, however, become unpopular or politically incorrect to present these calculations (see Chapter 7).

A revealing example of tension between overt and covert justification for screening comes from an area in Finland, where serum screening was established in the mid 1990s (Virkkula 1998). The political decision-makers were uncertain about the protocol, but became convinced after the clinical geneticist in charge had presented them with calculations of the costs of an individual with DS to society. There is nothing unique in such calculations, but the point here is that they were classified as confidential and became public only after research by a journalist. What followed was a heated discussion on the morality of screening for DS and calculating a price for human life. The clinical geneticist commented in the newspaper that it is easy to justify screening on medical grounds, but because political decision-makers understand only monetary issues, he had presented the calculations. It is not clear what he meant by 'medical grounds', but the statement seems to me to be another example of hidden common morality among the medical profession (see Chapter 5 on prenatal diagnosis).

Another cost is the rate of miscarriage after invasive procedures performed because of positive results in screening tests (Copel and Bahado-Singh 1999). As noted earlier in Chapter 5, such costs are related to both amniocentesis and chorionic villus sampling. The whole problem will vanish only if, in the future, it becomes possible to detect foetal cells from maternal blood.

Different screening policies yield different rates of true positives, false positives and adverse effects. Every policy involving invasive procedures brings about miscarriages of foetuses with normal chromosomes. The trade-offs of current policies have been recently analysed in an article in the *American Journal of Public Health* (Serra-Prat *et al.* 1998). The ratio of miscarriages to cases detected varied between 0.26 and 1.45, depending on the screening tools used and the cut-off point for the risk estimate above which diagnostic procedures were offered.

A third cost of screening is the emotional burden imposed on parents by false positive results. It is commonly acknowledged that pretest counselling is seldom adequate and that too many mothers-to-be have been ill-informed about the test. As Copel and Bahado-Singh (1999) have noted, 'We have often done a poor job of explaining the meaning of screening tests to parents-to-be and of clarifying that a low positive predictive value does not mean that a test is inaccurate'.

What is the rationale behind the cut-off point used in serum screening for DS? A common cut-off point has been a risk of 1 in 250. A calculated risk lower than 1 in 250 is considered low. Women whose risk is higher than 1 in 250 are offered definitive prenatal diagnosis. This cut-off point was originally selected for several reasons, all of which were not necessarily articulated explicitly.

Firstly, in the early days of prenatal diagnosis the resources for this activity were scarce, and wide use would have been out of the question (Kuppermann *et al.* 1999). Obviously, this is no longer a valid reason for justifying a cut-off point in developed countries.

Secondly, economic cost–benefit analyses performed in the 1970s were an important factor in defining the cut-off point for screening. Maternal age was originally the only criterion used, and it was concluded that offering amniocentesis to women 35 years and older would be cost-effective. Later, when serum screening was developed, the cut-off point of 1 in 250 was chosen because it roughly represents the risk of a 35-year-old woman. As noted, it is nowadays less common to refer to economic values when screening for DS is discussed. It is worth remembering, however, that earlier, one of the main justifications for the cut-off point still in use today was cost-related (Kent and Dornan 1996).

Thirdly, until the early 1970s, the birth prevalence data on DS were usually presented in 5-year risk intervals, and there seemed to be a sudden increase in risk at the age of 35 years. This age seemed thus to be a reasonable age threshold for offering invasive testing (Kuppermann *et al.* 1999). Later research showed, however, that the risk increases linearly between 20 and 30 years of age and then logarithmically beginning at about 33 years of age. Because there is no point at which the risk 'jumps' to a higher level, 35 years is, in this sense, as artificial as any other age (Kuppermann *et al.* 1999).

Fourthly, balancing the risks for foetal abnormality and for procedure-related miscarriage has been used as a justification for a cut-off point of 35 years of age for DS screening. Thirty-five years is the age at which the risk for a chromosomal abnormality in the foetus is roughly the same as the risk for miscarriage due to the prenatal diagnosis procedure (Kuppermann *et al.* 1999). After the introduction of serum screening the same logic has been used as justification for the cut-off point of 1 in 250.

There is an implicit assumption in this fourth justification that the women (or couples) in question would give equal weight to both outcomes. Empirical research shows that they do not (Kuppermann *et al.* 1999). According to a Californian study most women (83%) assigned a lower utility to having a child with Down syndrome than to experiencing a procedure-related miscarriage. On the other hand, there was substantial variation among women as to the preferences for these outcomes (Kuppermann *et al.* 1999). The researchers suggest that strict age- or risk-based cut-off points for determining the eligibility for prenatal diagnosis should be abandoned. Instead, prenatal diagnosis should be accessible to all women whose preferences indicate that such testing should be appropriate (Kuppermann *et al.* 1999).

Attitudes towards Down syndrome

The attitudes of medical professionals towards children with DS are far from uniform. In an interesting study, Wolraich *et al.* (1991) noted a difference between, for example, paediatric surgeons and paediatricians. The former gave significantly lower prognostications than the latter, when presented with two hypothetical cases. The authors also pointed out that doctors' prognostications of intellectually disabled individuals are lower than those of other professions and some are lower than actual outcomes (Wolraich *et al.* 1991). Since doctors are key actors in decision-making concerning these people, the consequences may be important.

Sometimes these consequences may be dramatic if the life of the child depends on an operation, as in the case of duodenal atresia. The following citation is from a report describing the legal investigation of one such case, in which the non-operated child died at the age of 17 days. The author, a paediatric surgeon, described the course of events and the legal process. The final paragraph represents, of course, his view alone and cannot be generalised to all paediatric surgeons:

> I firmly believe that, contrary to popular perception, a human being suffering from Down's syndrome alone is a tragedy and a cause of great suffering both to the particular human being and for his parents and family members. Medicine is the servant of mercy. (Molenaar 1992, p. 40)

There is also evidence of suboptimal medical care for some individuals with DS. A survey in Great Britain revealed that the vast majority gets good care but some do not. The syndrome has been used, for example, as justification for denying treatment for hearing or sight problems (Mayor 1999). A study in France reported an excess of unexplained deaths among children with DS but no known malformation (Julian-Reynier *et al.* 1995), and an American study found 16 children with DS who had received bone marrow transplants during a time when the expected number of such children would have been 63. The authors discussed several explanations, including parental refusal based on a physician's advice (Arenson and Forde 1989).

Why should Down syndrome be prevented?

In the previous chapter I discussed arguments that have been presented to support the prevention of ID. These arguments were (1) the eugenic argument, (2) the foetal-wastage argument, (3) the family burden argument, (4) the societal burden argument and (5) the quality of life argument.

The first two arguments were shown to be vague and weak, and now I shall consider only the latter three arguments and their relevance to DS.

What can be said about the burden on families with a child with DS? In fact a lot, since empirical research has been conducted in several countries to address the issue. The general impression is that most families adapt well in their life with a member with DS (Bränholm and Degerman 1992, Carr 1995). However, some families have great problems, which make them especially vulnerable. There are also research results that may help to identify these vulnerable families (Gath 1990).

Obviously great variation exists in parental attitudes towards their offspring with DS. Maybe the words of a mother summarise the experience in most families. When asked about her opinion on abortion after amniocentesis, she replied:

> If I hadn't already had one it would be an easier decision but I've had W and she is classed as handicapped. But she's lovely, she seems as normal as can be, so I couldn't have an abortion after W, but if I hadn't had her, my idea of *being* handicapped would be different. (Shepperdson 1983, p. 153)

Another issue that has been researched in families has been the influence of a child with DS on the well-being of siblings. Here, too, the general impression is normality in sibling interaction (Carr 1995).

The economic consequences of having a child with DS do not differ from those of having an intellectually disabled child in general. As noted in Chapter 7, they are highly dependent on the way health and social services are arranged.

The societal burden argument can refer to either economic or other costs of DS to society in general. In fact, screening for DS was shown to be cost-effective very early after the introduction of methods for prenatal screening. The cut-off point for high or low risk (usually 1/250) still in use today was determined by the early cost–benefit analyses in the 1970s (Kent and Dornan 1996). Thus the economic justification for this screening has not disappeared although other values are nowadays emphasised.

The non-economic burdens of DS on society are more difficult to grasp. Even in utilitarian terms it is not obvious that the amount of happiness created by a screening system is greater than the amount of happiness without such a system. If the general impression of persons with DS as joyful and positive is true, aborting foetuses with DS may in fact decrease the total happiness of a future world. Of course, these kinds of statements are too speculative and, possibly all that can be reliably said is that we cannot determine the cost-effectiveness of screening in terms of happiness achieved.

The last argument considered here is the quality of life argument. I did not find studies that would have directly compared the quality of life with DS to life without it. One can also question the validity of such an approach. Aspects of Having and Loving (see Chapter 7) would be easier to compare, but aspects of Being would be more or less associated with intellectual performance. If questionnaires were used to measure quality of life, the group with DS would at least partly be represented by parents or educators.

The lack of such comparative data does not mean that nothing can be said about the quality of life of people with DS. Anecdotal evidence tells a lot. Comparative studies have been done among persons with DS, and the studies on family life describe indirectly the lives of the members with DS. First, two very different stories.

Susanna and Tomi are a married couple, rare because they never argue, unique because they both have DS. They live quite ordinary lives: go to work, watch television and listen to music in the evenings, go swimming and fight against going overweight. They do not pay taxes because they go to a sheltered workshop, and they are also visited weekly by a social worker. Both Susanna and Tomi can read and also write and calculate a little. Their favourite television programme is *The Bold and the Beautiful* (Palo 1995).

Another story is anonymous, and it was presented in an article describing a study on the views of parents of children with DS on abortion and euthanasia. One mother said:

If I knew as I know now I'd have euthanasiaed [*sic*] her. It's cruel for me and cruel for her. There's no life for me while she's here and none for her . . . it's not a bit of good, the country's better off without them . . . a handicapped mind and a handicapped body, it's cruel. When a dog's injured you put it down. (Shepperdson 1983, p. 154)

We do not know why the mother in the latter story felt so miserable. Maybe her daughter had diseases or physical handicaps associated with DS. Maybe the family received little or no social support. Maybe the daughter had especially low intelligence. Comparative studies show that adults with DS in family care are better oriented, more skilled and productive and emotionally stable and less disturbed than institutionalised adults with DS.

Studies on the quality of life in families with a member with DS have already been described. Their lives do not differ very much from the lives of other families. There is no reason to assume that the quality of life of the individual with DS would, in general, be very different from the rest of the family.

Why, then, should DS be prevented? The family burden and quality of life arguments have not turned out to give strong *general* support for the prevention of DS. Of course there may be vulnerable families in which the birth of a child with DS would bring about a burden extremely hard to bear. This statement cannot, however, be generalised to the claim that DS should *always* be prevented.

People with DS are a burden to society, at least in economic terms. In that sense the interest of society would be to have as few people with DS as possible. In the early 1970s compulsory screening was suggested, but it has, to my knowledge, never taken place. Reproductive autonomy has been considered a value that cannot be overridden by economics.

The medical discourse on prenatal screening for and diagnosis of DS has been dominated by issues like 'where the cut-off point should be set'; 'what an acceptable risk for procedure-related miscarriage is' or 'what the uptake of the screening test is'. The main question, however, is 'what should be done about Down syndrome' (Lippman 1999). Prenatal diagnosis is one, but just one, possible answer. True reproductive autonomy means true choice for women and couples, and it includes full support also for those who reject testing or decide to continue pregnancy even if what is looked for during the testing is found.

One way towards enhanced autonomy would be to abandon age- or risk-based cut-off points for determining the eligibility for prenatal diagnosis. As in the current systems, women would first choose whether to participate in screening at all. Those who would decide to be tested would then make their own decisions according to the test results and their own values. Of course, this system would necessitate extensive counselling, and the resources may not meet the demand in many societies. In Philip Kitcher's words: 'the transition to societies in which genetic testing is more prevalent will almost certainly multiply the number of situations in which "respecting the autonomy of the counseled" would be a bitter joke' (Kitcher 1997, pp. 78–9).

In practice, a mid-way solution could be something like the present system in a South Wales district in the UK, where the screening practices for DS were standardised and improved in the late 1990s (Al-Jader 1999). The starting point for the quality improvement process was an earlier report that had identified substandard and variable practices. One of the keystones of the development process was that the opinions and the expectations of expectant mothers were asked. As a result of the whole process, the uptake of serum screening *fell* from around 95% to 75%. In addition, the number of amniocenteses decreased as women were able to think more clearly about their options and the limitations of the tests (Al-Jader 1999).

Fragile X syndrome

It was noted about 100 years ago that ID is commoner among men than among women. In 1943 Martin and Bell described sex-linked inheritance of intellectual disability in a family, and the cause of that disability was later called fragile X syndrome (fraX). This took place in the late 1970s when a fragile site in the X chromosome of these people was found. The gene responsible for fraX was discovered in 1991 and DNA testing soon became possible (Peippo 1995, Murray *et al.* 1997).

FraX is caused by an abnormally high number of consecutive repeating cytosine–guanine–guanine (CGG) triplets in the DNA of the gene labelled FMR-1. The genotype is classified as normal, premutational or full mutational, based on the number of these triplets (Palomaki 1994). In the unaffected population the average number of these triplets is 30, in premutation they number from about 55 to 199 and in full mutation there are 200 or more (Murray *et al.* 1997). Full mutation is associated with clinical fraX, and premutation carries a high risk of expansion between mother and offspring. Other defects in the FMR-1 gene are also possible, but they are thought to be rare (Murray *et al.* 1997).

The association between full mutation and the fraX phenotype differs for men and women. Nearly all males with full mutation have the fraX phenotype, but only half of females with full mutation have the genotype with learning disabilities, one fifth having a moderate to severe phenotype (Murray *et al.* 1997).

FraX is inherited as an X-linked disorder, but the inheritance pattern is not similar as in classic X-linked recessive disorders. In the latter, females are carriers and only males are affected. With fraX, both can be affected, although females to a less extent (Murray *et al.* 1997). In addition, both males and females can be unaffected carriers. The children of unaffected female carriers are at increased risk of the disorder, but children of unaffected male carriers are not (Murray *et al.* 1997).

The latter, so-called 'normal transmitting males', have sons that are neither affected nor carriers, while all their daughters are unaffected carriers. The children of these daughters are at increased risk of the syndrome.

Characteristics

FraX is characterised by a mixture of physical, cognitive and behavioural features. General physical health is not impaired, although fraX is manifested in many organ systems. The affected males have a typical facial appearance, orthopaedic abnormalities, skin manifestations, cardiac anomalies and endocrine dysfunction (Murray *et al.* 1997).

About 80% of the males are moderately to severely intellectually disabled with IQs of less than 50. Most females with fraX have borderline IQs between 70 and 85 (Murray *et al.* 1997).

There is no specific therapy for fraX, but there are several medical, educational, psychological and social interventions that can improve the symptoms (Murray *et al.* 1997).

Epidemiology

It is difficult to estimate the prevalence of fraX in populations because, for a reliable estimate, a very large sample of people would have to be tested. Another difficulty concerns the diagnostic methodology. After the introduction of DNA-based diagnosis the older cytogenetic methods were found to produce false positive results (Murray *et al.* 1997).

However, several studies have been performed, mainly testing young people with special educational needs. On the basis of these studies, Murray *et al.* (1997) estimated that the minimum prevalence is 1 per 4000 among males and 1 per 8000 among females.

Prevention

Because no specific treatment exists for fraX, primary prevention is possible only by identifying females at high risk of an affected pregnancy. Once these women are found there are several options: prenatal diagnosis and selective abortion, avoidance of pregnancy, in vitro fertilisation of a donated ovum and preimplantation diagnosis (Murray *et al.* 1997).

Identifying females at risk could take place in three ways. Firstly, a preconceptual screening programme could target, for example, school leavers or attendees at family planning clinics (Murray *et al.* 1997). Secondly, prenatal screening could be offered to pregnant women with the possibility for prenatal diagnosis for those testing positive. Thirdly, in so-called 'cascade screening', the relatives of an affected individual could be offered counselling and DNA testing.

Ethical issues

Why, then, should fraX be prevented? A response to the general arguments presented for prevention is essentially similar to that in the case of DS. Most people with fraX are an economic burden to society. With respect to the family burden and quality of life arguments, there is no *general* justification for prevention.

The process for screening for fraX differs, however, from that of screening for DS, and there are some ethical issues unique to the prevention of fraX.

Serum or ultrasound screening for DS yields a risk figure only, and the definitive diagnosis is possible only after an invasive diagnostic procedure. DNA testing of the mother definitively describes *her* status with respect to fraX: non-affected, premutation or full mutation. In the first case her offspring will have no risk for fraX. Only if the father were a normal transmitting male, would possible daughters in this family have an increased risk for sons with fraX.

In the second case the foetus is at increased risk for fraX, the risk being greater for male than female foetuses. In the third case the mother may be unaffected or herself have some, usually minor manifestations of fraX. For her foetuses the risk would be similar to the second case.

I have already mentioned two examples of the ethical complexity of inheritance in families with fraX (see Chapter 5 on prenatal diagnosis). In the first a clinical geneticist was talking about the difficulties of counselling in cases in which one relative had fraX. When describing a particular case of a healthy pregnant woman with the fragile X genotype, the geneticist said: 'It would be hard to make her understand why, *according to the view of modern medicine*, a foetus with the same genotype as the mother, should be aborted . . .'.

The event took place about ten years ago. When I recently described it to another clinical geneticist in Finland, she replied that today such comments would not be heard. However, the case serves as an example of hidden values in clinical decision-making and the uncertainty which pregnant women still have to face in actual practice.

In the second case a pregnant young woman with a retarded brother with fraX discussed her feelings of whether she would have chosen abortion if her first test had shown the syndrome. She was ambivalent but said that she would not necessarily want an abortion in such a case. Because of her experiences with her brother, and taking care of him, she did not feel it to be such a terrible burden.

It is easy, of course, to imagine another example, in which a pregnant woman has had very negative experiences with a brother with fraX. Maybe she would be convinced that she would have a male foetus with fraX aborted.

The parental uncertainty in screening for fraX is thus different from that in screening for DS. If the mother is found to be a carrier of fraX, either premutation or full mutation, the parents have to make the first decision: whether or not go on to invasive testing. If the foetus is tested and found to have fraX, the parents then have to face the uncertainty of the prognosis.

In the medical literature the problem is sometimes addressed straightforwardly. The ethical dilemma concerns only or mainly cases in which the foetus is female. For example Palomaki (1994, p. 69), has written:

> … the inability to distinguish which of the female foetuses with a full mutation fragile X genotype will be affected represents a serious ethical dilemma for the medical community and for the pregnant woman. Given this constraint, implementing fragile X screening would mean that nearly half of all women with a foetus identified as having a full mutation could be faced with making reproductive decisions based on only a 50% likelihood of the foetus being affected. It is mainly for this reason that it is difficult to argue strongly in favour of initiating population based screening for fragile X at this time.

There are two hidden messages here. Firstly, there are no major ethical issues in screening for fraX when the foetus is known to be male. Secondly, if the likelihood of a female foetus would not be 50% but, say, 95%, the ethical problems would be considerably fewer.

What seems problematic to me is the assumption that it is up to the medical community to decide what likelihood is high enough to justify screening. While it is true that medical research tells us about the percentages, the conclusions drawn are based on value judgements in which the medical community can not claim authority over the families involved.

Preconceptual screening would eliminate the anxiety which prenatal screening easily provokes. However, few women take part in screening if it is offered pre-conceptually. Prenatal screening reaches a far greater percentage of women at risk. However, the question of the aim of screening should be asked again. If the aim is to reduce the birth prevalence of fraX, the obvious aim should be an uptake of 100%.

If, on the other hand, the aim is to offer families information for their own reproductive choices, an uptake of 100% raises questions about the validity of the counselling and consent processes. An obvious analogy would be a country in which the voting percentage is 100%. An uptake of 85% (which was reached in a study in Kuopio, Finland) shows that at least minimally satisfactory freedom of decision was reached. If the real aim is to provide information, the uptake is in the end irrelevant and the success of the process should be measured in other terms.

Aspartylglucosaminuria

AGU (aspartylglucosaminuria) is a recessively inherited lysosomal storage disor-der caused by mutations in the aspartylglucosaminidase gene on chromosome 4

(Isoniemi *et al.* 1995). It is strongly concentrated in the population of Finland. Over 200 patients have been identified there in contrast to approximately 40 cases in the rest of the world (Hietala *et al.* 1993).

AGU was first described in the late 1960s, and the concentration of it in the Finnish population was reported in 1970. Estimations of the carrier frequency in Finland are in the range of 1 : 30 to 1 : 80 (Hietala 1998). Because AGU is a recessive disorder, the number of actual cases is, however, small.

Characteristics

The progress of AGU is very slow. The prenatal period and early infancy are often uneventful, but recurrent infections and hernias may occur more often than in the general population. Usually the first sign of the disease itself is a delay or arrest in speech development (Hietala 1998). Mental delay then progresses slowly through childhood and adolescence, and typical physical characteristics like a coarse face appear. The degree of ID in adulthood is severe, but in spite of the accumulation of abnormal degradation products in many organs there are no obvious functional disturbances outside the central nervous system (Hietala 1998).

The average life span of AGU patients in a large Finnish study was 37.6 years (Arvio 1993), but the oldest reported patient has lived up to 69 years of age (Hietala 1998).

There is no specific therapy for AGU. However, a trial with bone marrow transplantation (BMT) is in progress (Autti *et al.* 1997). Early histopathological, biochemical and radiological findings supported the success of the transplantation, but the clinical follow-up of the patients could not demonstrate improvement (Arvio *et al.* 2001).

Prevention

As with fraX, current possibilities for the primary prevention of AGU are based on the identification of carriers. Once the carriers are found the following options are available: avoiding pregnancy, selecting a spouse who is not a carrier, in vitro fertilisation of a donated ovum (in the case of a female carrier), artificial insemination by a donor (in the case of a male carrier), prenatal diagnosis and termination of affected pregnancies and, at least in theory, preimplantation diagnosis.

Selecting partners on the basis of a gene test result is, of course, a powerful strategy in prevention. It has, in fact, proved to be successful in the prevention of Tay–Sachs disease, another lysosomal storage disorder, among orthodox Jews (Hietala 1998). A prerequisite for such a prevention programme is a community in which marriages are arranged by families, thus allowing the consideration of the gene test results.

In most Western societies today, however, the autonomy of adults is considered a trumping value, which cannot be overridden by community interests. In addition, the termination of affected pregnancies is widely considered an acceptable option. Among non-orthodox Jews, many of whom accept abortion due to a serious disease like Tay–Sachs, screening through prenatal diagnosis and selective termination has also been very successful. This success has been based on wide co-operation between medical practitioners, community leaders and religious leaders (Hietala 1998).

Identifying carriers could take place in many ways. Testing could take place in high schools, it could be offered in the basic health care system for people of a certain age or as part of maternity care during pregnancy. Much of the research in this area has concerned cystic fibrosis, which is the commonest severe autosomal recessive disorder among populations of northern European origin. Many pilot studies have been done, but so far no country has established a continuing screening programme. However, a consensus statement of the National Institutes of Health in the USA has recommended the offering of a carrier test for cystic fibrosis to couples planning a pregnancy or seeking prenatal care (Hietala 1998).

If screening takes place before pregnancy, an obvious advantage is that the couple's reproductive choices are informed concerning the particular trait screened for. The problem is that actual participation rates in non-pregnant populations have been markedly lower than for screening during pregnancy (Hietala 1988).

Screening during pregnancy can be sequential or couple screening. In the former the woman is tested first and her husband or partner is tested only if she proves to be a carrier. In the latter strategy samples are taken from both parents at the same time.

Carrier screening for AGU has been carried out in two pilot studies in Finland. The first took place in Helsinki between 1994 and 1995, and AGU carrier screening was used as a model with which to evaluate the feasibility of a genetic screening programme in primary health care (Hietala 1998). The general conclusions of the study were that such a programme can be successfully implemented in primary health maternity care and that the Finnish population in general and the family members of AGU patients in particular had mainly positive attitudes toward genetic testing. Because of the rarity of AGU the author suggested that multiplex screening for several disease genes should be considered instead of screening for AGU alone.

The second study was conducted in Kuopio from 1995 to 1996, when pregnant women were offered carrier screening for AGU, fraX and infantile neuronal ceroid lipofuscinosis (INCL), which is another rare recessive disease concentrated in Finland. The project created tension between the researchers and the health care authorities, and it was ended sooner than was planned. The reasons for the closure were complex, but the questionability of informed choice was a main consideration (Jallinoja 2001).

Ethical issues

The general ethical aspects of the prevention of AGU resemble those already discussed in the context of DS and fraX. Having a child with AGU in the family will no doubt eventually turn out to be a burden sooner or later. During infancy years, however, the life of the family is probably no different from the life of an average family. The progressive clinical course of AGU increases the family burden, at least in terms of a lack of independence of the AGU individual. If the correct diagnosis is obtained in early childhood, which obviously is the case at least in Finland, where the disease is known, the future course of the disease and also the burden on the family can be predicted.

The societal burden of AGU is small due to its rarity. Of course, individuals with AGU will never become good tax-payers, but, on the other hand, they usually spend their childhood years at home with their parents and are able to attend sheltered workshops in adulthood.

As with DS and fraX, the quality of life argument is weak in that the quality of life of people with AGU does not, as such, support a general prevention programme.

Should screening for AGU, then, be included as a part of prenatal screening offered in Finland? Or should corresponding recessive conditions be screened for in other parts of the world?

The conclusion of the study by Hietala *et al.* (1993) was that multiplex screening for several disease genes should be considered instead of screening for AGU alone. The general attitudes towards such testing are mainly positive and the attitudes of the families of AGU patients have proved to be especially positive. The experiences in the experimental screening project in Kuopio showed, however, that very complex ethical issues arise. If, say, 10 or 15 recessive genes are tested in one package and this test is offered as part of standard maternity care, it is highly unlikely that the families involved are well-enough informed about all the conditions and what follows if one or more of the results are positive. This is not to say that such tests should not be developed and that such testing should never take place. Those interested should have access to knowledge about their genes, but before any general system is built up into maternity care or elsewhere, there should be enough resources for adequate counselling before, during and after the testing.

10

Conclusion

At the beginning of this book I presented four cases. Now it is time to return to these cases and draw some conclusions. But first, a brief summary of the case presentations.

In Case 1 Sarah and Tom have just heard the results of the serum screening test, according to which Sarah's risk for carrying a foetus with Down syndrome is 1 in 150. Now they have to decide whether they wish to have an accurate diagnosis by amniocentesis, which, however, increases slightly the risk of miscarriage. The nurse at the maternity clinic is sympathetic but refuses to answer Sarah's question about how she would decide if she were in a similar situation.

In Case 2 Tina and Harry are expecting their first child. Tina has a younger brother who has fragile X syndrome and is mildly intellectually disabled. Tina is a carrier of the syndrome and knows that the probability for intellectual disability in her possible future offspring is considerable. Tina is more positive than Harry about the idea of continuing pregnancy with a male foetus with fragile X syndrome.

The first two cases were fictional, although they could very well be true. Case 3 is real and takes us from the individual to the community level: How should health authorities in eastern and northern Finland respond to the suggestion that testing for the AGU (aspartylglucosaminuria) gene were introduced to routine maternity care?

Case 4 is also real, and, in fact, it is a very famous one. The fate of Baby Jane Doe, a child with Down syndrome and oesophageal atresia, created much controversy in the USA in the 1980s. There was nothing very specific in the case as such. It is highly probable that many children with a similar condition have faced similar death on both sides of the Atlantic. The disagreement between doctors and the early involvement of courts of law were probably the main factors that made the case so well known.

Definition

In Chapter 2, I discussed in detail the definition of intellectual disability (ID) and many related issues. In light of that discussion, what can be said about cases 1–4 and the foetuses or children involved?

According to definition 1 'a person is intellectually disabled if he or she falls below two standard deviations in a standardised intelligence test'. In light of this definition, the probability for ID would be very high in cases 1 and 4, Down syndrome. In case 3, AGU, the affected individuals definitely end up being intellectually disabled, but it would happen only after relatively normal first years of life. In case 2 the prognosis would be the most uncertain: a boy with fragile X genotype could be severely, moderately or mildly intellectually disabled or have normal intelligence.

Definition 2 paints a more colourful picture of ID, and, in addition, subaverage intellectual functioning refers to 'related limitations in two or more of the following applicable adaptive skill areas: communication, self-care, home living, social skills, community use, self-direction, health and safety, functional academics, leisure and work'. It is, however, obvious that this definition would cover my cases in a manner that closely resembles that of definition 1. Some individuals with Down syndrome may be quite independent in their lives, but extremely few would not have limitations in less than two of the areas mentioned.

Epidemiology

In cases 1, 2 and 4 individual families faced difficult decisions about abortion or quality of life or both. In case 1 the family was involved in a screening programme, in case 2 the problem could be anticipated because of the family history, and in case 4 the problem became obvious only after the birth of the child and the diagnosis of oesophageal atresia.

Down syndrome and fragile X syndrome are the commonest genetic causes of intellectual disability, and especially screening for the former has been a hot topic in biomedical research for over two decades. It should be remembered, however, that people with these syndromes are still a minority among the intellectually disabled. Even if there were available screening methods with 100% sensitivity and specificity and if every foetus with these syndromes were aborted, the impact on the general prevalence of ID would be less than 20%. And, as has become obvious, this is a highly improbable scenario for both scientific and ethical reasons.

Case 3 focused on the level of society, and the burden of decision was on the health authorities. Of course, if screening is introduced, the burden is on individuals, as in the other cases. From the point of view of epidemiology the significance of the decision is almost nil in any case. The whole question of screening for the AGU gene is worth bringing up only for certain parts of Finland, and even in these areas only occasional cases of ID could be prevented even with a 100% uptake of tests.

Prenatal diagnosis and screening

Case 1, 2 and 3 demonstrate most of the ethical issues mentioned in Chapter 5 on prenatal diagnosis and screening. Firstly, the issue of the consent of parents does not seem to be a problem in cases 1 and 2 (and it is as yet irrelevant in case 3). According to the case descriptions both the couple with a 1 : 150 risk for Down syndrome and the couple with possible fragile X offspring seemed well informed. The former couple consented to screening and the latter was considering the possibility of prenatal diagnosis.

Secondly, the tension between the reproductive autonomy model and the public health model is obvious in cases 1 and 3. Although it is common in the rhetoric of today's medicine to state that screening programmes exist to enhance the reproductive autonomy of individual women and families, there is no doubt that a public health perspective exists there too. The risk for Down syndrome in case 1 was 1 : 150, and it was considered 'high'. Someone had decided that the risk was high enough to justify the offer of an invasive procedure. Although not obvious today, it is plausible that cost–benefit calculations from the early years of prenatal screening still influence the cut-off points used today. In case 3 it is also obvious that screening for AGU is not considered solely for the reproductive autonomy of individual families. If it were so, it would be totally irrelevant whether or not the families who screen positive opt for abortion.

Thirdly, in case 2, the possibility of a prenatal diagnosis can be seen as a response to a request from the woman (couple). With a long experience of life in a fragile X family, she is a true expert on the social and psychological aspects of the syndrome. Her request, if anybody's, can be thought of as justified. This kind of case may, however, be an exception in the context of prenatal diagnosis and screening. It may be that the availability of screening technology has created the request and not vice versa.

Fourthly, reassurance is a relevant issue in cases 1, 2 and 3. Most women who undergo prenatal diagnostic testing receive good news (although the good news of not having the condition sought for is too often interpreted as news of a healthy foetus). The probability for Down syndrome in case 1 is very small and the probability for AGU (if the screening is introduced) in case 3 is even smaller. In case 2 the probability for an intellectually disabled offspring is high, but the issue of reassurance is still relevant.

Fifthly, the question of eugenics, 'deliberate control, by law or social pressure, of the perpetuation of human genetic traits', is worth mentioning briefly. Such control of reproduction by law is obviously out of the question in Western democracies.

Case 3 describes, however, a situation, which may introduce social pressure. Although there have been only experimental studies on AGU screening, empirical evidence from other existing programmes has demonstrated that such social pressure can be real.

Genetic counselling

Did genetic counselling take place and was it successful in our cases?

In case 1 there was no formal genetic counselling in the sense that a genetic counsellor would have been involved. Nevertheless, the couple seemed to have been well informed by their maternity clinic personnel, who described Down syndrome briefly and gave the parents a leaflet about it. On a later occasion the nurse refused to answer Sarah's question about how she would decide in a similar situation. She was, however sympathetic and promised to give her full support, whatever the decision. At least superficially the course of events seems satisfactory. From the case description it can be inferred that the couple did not take for granted any of the alternatives. The decision to take part in the screening was made freely and although we do not know whether amniocentesis was performed, at least the couple was well informed of the situation.

From the point of view of genetic counselling, case 2 seems simple, since Tina had inside knowledge about fragile X syndrome and had already been tested and found to be a carrier. The case is, however, simple only if genetic counselling is mainly thought of as counselling about *facts*. There would be an obvious role here for dialogical counselling, 'ensuring that decisions are as fully informed and carefully deliberated as possible' (White 1999). A good genetic counsellor could help the couple in a 'joint search for a morally excusable decision' (Hoedemaekers 1998).

In light of studies performed in Finland, it is not probable that, in case 3, health authorities will decide to introduce AGU screening in maternity care. The main reason for this attitude would be the rarity of the disease, but perhaps multiplex screening for AGU *and* some other diseases would be suggested instead. As noted at the end of Chapter 9, this decision would, however, create an almost untenable situation from the point of view of genetic counselling.

If the case descriptions concerning Baby Doe, case 4, are truthful, obviously no adequate genetic counselling took place. We do not know what kind of information was provided by the obstetrician and the paediatricians involved, but Baby Doe's father hardly would have talked about the 'never ... a minimally acceptable quality of life' after even minimal counselling about the facts of Down syndrome. Whatever the final decision of the parents, 'ensuring that decisions are as fully informed and carefully deliberated as possible' would have been better.

It is, of course, obvious that, in the cases demonstrated, Down syndrome, fragile X syndrome and AGU, genes determine, to a high degree, the lives of these individuals. Thus one might be tempted to think that geneticisation does not play a role here: what is genetic is genetic period.

However, geneticisation and genetic determinism are relevant also in the context of cases like these. An individual is, after all, a product of both genes and the environment, even in a case in which genes radically limit the potential for intellectual development. The genes may determine the upper limit of intellectual capacity in Down syndrome and fragile X syndrome and the speed of deterioration in AGU, but this determination does not mean that various forms of therapy would have no or only minor influence on the lives of these people. In addition, the strong position of genetics in the world of science means that research aiming at, for example, enhancing communication skills among the intellectually disabled is in a much weaker position than biological research is.

Why prevent?

The reasons for preventing ID were discussed generally in Chapter 7 and with respect to Down syndrome, fragile X syndrome and AGU in Chapter 9.

The eugenic argument and the foetal-wastage argument proved weak and vague, and they are not considered here. The societal burden argument, the family burden argument and the quality of life argument are briefly reviewed with respect to the cases.

Although cost–benefit calculations may never be very accurate in the context of prenatal screening, there is no doubt that most people with Down syndrome (case 1) or AGU (case 3) are an economic burden to society. The situation is less clear with fragile X syndrome (case 2) since the spectrum of intelligence is wide and not all individuals are intellectually disabled. As a group, however, people with fragile X can be said to be an economic burden to society. Thus it would be in the interest of society to prevent these syndromes.

The non-economic burdens to society are far less obvious. In fact, even the opposite can take place and a 'burden' can turn into something else. A paediatrician with long experience in the field of ID wrote recently that people with Down syndrome are 'the elite among the intellectually disabled, who usually live a happy life and enrich the environment with their joyfulness' (Wilska 2001). It is, of course, as difficult or impossible to quantify this kind of enrichment as it is to quantify the emotional burden in these families. In real life some families with an intellectually disabled child do well while others do not.

The burdens on individual families with an intellectually disabled child can take different forms, psychological and economic. They vary substantially and should be dealt with in the context of society and the health care system. There is no evidence of substantial burdens that ruin the lives of these families *generally*. However, in *particular* cases, having a child with Down syndrome, fragile X or AGU may be a terrible burden to the rest of the family. If abortion on request is accepted and if parental autonomy in reproductive issues is valued highly, then it is up to Sarah and Tom (case 1) and Tina and Harry (case 2) to decide whether the expected burden in their families is great enough to justify abortion.

While the family burden argument refers to the life of other individuals in the family, the quality of life argument concerns the individual with ID. Although there are problems with the concept of quality of life, it is not obvious that the quality of life in Down syndrome (case 1 and 4), the fragile X syndrome (case 2) or AGU (case 3) would be considerably lower than that in the general population. Existing empirical evidence shows that differences are minor. In addition, quality of life is so much determined by external factors that it may not be meaningful to refer to whole groups of people with these syndromes, especially when physical handicaps usually play a minor role in the lives of these individuals.

Moral status

In Chapter 8, I presented Mary Ann Warren's multi-criterial theory of moral status and applied it to potential or actual individuals with or without ID.

In cases 1 and 2 we had two young foetuses, who, according to the Respect of Life principle, had some moral status and should not be killed or otherwise harmed, without good reasons that do not violate the other principles. They were not yet sentient, and therefore the Anti-Cruelty principle was not valid. The mothers (families) had full moral status, and, if a conflict of interest between the foetuses and the mothers (families) would have arisen, abortion may have been justified. ID as such would not lower the moral status of foetuses under these circumstances, but it may be a contributing factor when mothers (families) make decisions about their future.

In case 4 the situation was different. According to the Human Rights principle, Baby Doe should have had the same moral rights as moral agents have, within the limits of her own capacities and the limits of the Agent's Rights principle. Baby Doe's oesophageal atresia was certainly relevant in the case, but her Down syndrome was relevant only if it could be shown to have an effect on her *physical* prognosis. ID in relation to Down syndrome should not have had an effect on her care.

References

Abramowicz, H. K., Richardson, S. A. 1975. Epidemiology of severe mental retardation in children: community studies. *Am. J. Ment. Defic.* 80: 18–39.

Al-Jader, L. 1999. The achievements of antenatal screening programme for congenital abnormalities and lessons learned for clinical governance. *J. Med. Genet.* 36 (Suppl. 1): S70.

Allardt, E. 1993. Having, Loving, Being: An alternative to the Swedish model of welfare research. In: Nussbaum, M. C., Sen, A. (Eds) *The Quality of Life*, pp. 88–94. Oxford: Clarendon Press.

American Association on Mental Retardation 1992. *Mental Retardation: Definition, Classification and Systems of Supports, 9th edn.* Washington, DC: American Association on Mental Retardation.

Arenson, E. B., Forde, M. D. 1989. Bone marrow transplantation for acute leukemia and Down syndrome: report of a successful case and results of a national survey. *J. Pediatr.* 114: 69–72.

Arvio, M. 1993. *Life with Aspartylglucosaminuria* (Dissertation). Pääjärvi Rehabilitation Centre and Department of Child Neurology, University of Helsinki, Finland.

Arvio, M., Sauna-Aho, O., Peippo, M. 2001. Bone marrow transplantation for aspartylglucosaminuria: follow-up study of transplanted and non-transplanted patients. *J. Pediatr.* 138: 288–90.

Autti, T., Santavuori, P., Raininko, R., Renlund, M., Rapola, J., Saarinen-Pihkala, U. 1997. Bone-marrow transplantation in aspartylglucosaminuria. *Lancet* 349: 1366–7.

Bahado-Singh, R., Shahabi, S., Karaca, M., Mahoney, M. J., Cole, L., Oz, U. A. 2002. The comprehensive midtrimester test: high-sensitivity Down syndrome test. *Am. J. Obstet. Gynecol.* 186: 803–8.

Baird, P. A., Sadovnick, A. D. 1988. Life expectancy in Down syndrome adults. *Lancet* ii: 1354–6.

Behrman, R. E., Vaughan, V. C. (Eds) 1987. *Nelson Textbook of Pediatrics, 13th edn.* Philadelphia, PA: W. B. Saunders.

Benjamin, J., Li, L., Patterson, C., Greenberg, B. D., Murphy, D. L., Hamer, D. H. 1996. Population and familial association between the D4 dopamine receptor gene and measures of Novelty Seeking. *Nat. Genet.* 12(Jan): 81–4.

Berger, M., Yule, W. 1985. IQ test and assessment. In: Clarke, A. M., Clarke, D. B., Berg, J. M. (Eds) *Mental Deficiency: The Changing Outlook*, pp. 53–95. Cambridge: Methuen and Co.

Bianchi, D. W. 1995. Prenatal diagnosis by analysis of fetal cells in maternal blood. *J. Pediatr.* 127: 847–56.

Block, N. J., Dworkin, G. 1974. IQ, Heritability and Inequality, Part 1. *Philos. Public Affairs* 3: 331–409.

1975. IQ, Heritability and Inequality, Part 2. *Philos. Public Affairs* 4: 40–99.

Boddington, P., Podpadec, T. 1991. Who are the mentally handicapped? *J. Appl. Philos.* 8: 177–90.

Boorse, C. 1975. On the distinction between disease and illness. *Philos. Public Affairs* 5: 49–68.

Booth, B. E., Verma, M., Singh Beri, R. 1994. Fetal sex determination in Punjab, India: correlations and implications. *Br. Med. J.* 309: 1259–61.

Booth, T. 1985. Labels and their consequences. In: Lane, D., Stratford, B. (Eds) *Current Approaches to Down's syndrome*, pp. 3–24. Eastbourne: Holt, Rinehart and Winston.

Borthwick-Duffy, S. A. 1996. Evaluation and measurement of quality of life: special considerations for persons with mental retardation. In: Schalock, R. L., Siperstein, G. N. (Eds) *Quality of Life Volume I. Conceptualization and Measurement*, pp. 105–19. Washington, DC: American Association on Mental Retardation.

Bosk, C. L. 1992. *All God's Mistakes. Genetic Counseling in a Pediatric Hospital.* Chicago: The University of Chicago Press.

Boss, J. A. 1990. How voluntary prenatal diagnosis and selective abortion increase the abnormal human gene pool. *Birth* 17: 75–9.

1993. *The Birth Lottery. Prenatal Diagnosis and Selective Abortion.* Chicago: Loyola University Press.

Bouchard, L., Renaud, M. 1997. Female and male physicians' attitudes toward prenatal diagnosis: a pan-Canadian survey. *Soc. Sci. Med.* 44: 381–92.

Bourguignon, H. J. 1994. Mental retardation: the reality behind the label. *Camb. Q. Health. Ethics* 3: 179–94.

Brambati, B., Formigli, L., Tului, L., Simoni, G. 1990. Selective reduction of quadruplet pregnancy at risk of Beta-thalassemia. *Lancet* 336: 1325–6.

Bränholm, I. B., Degerman, E. A. 1992. Life satisfaction and activity preferences in parents of Down's syndrome children. *Scand. J. Soc. Med.* 20: 37–44.

Brøndum-Nielsen, K., Nørgaard-Pedersen, B. 1993. Prenatal diagnostik i Norden. *Nordisk Medicin.* 108: 189–92.

Burleigh, M. 1994. *Death and Deliverance. 'Euthanasia' in Germany 1900–1945.* Cambridge: Cambridge University Press.

Burton, L. 1975. *The Family Life of Sick Children.* London: Routledge and Kegan Paul.

Cairney, R. 1996. Democracy was never intended for degenerates: Alberta's flirtation with eugenics comes back to haunt it. *Can. Med. Assoc. J.* 155: 789–92.

Callahan, D. 1996. The genetic revolution. In: Thomasma, D., Kushner, T. (Eds) *Birth to Death. Science and Bioethics*, pp. 13–20. Cambridge: Cambridge University Press.

Campbell, A. V. 1984. Ethical issues in prenatal diagnosis. *Br. Med. J. Clin. Res. Ed.* 288: 1633–4.

Canguilhem, G. 1978. *On the Normal and the Pathological.* Dordrecht: Reidel.

Carr, J. 1995. *Down's Syndrome Children Growing up.* Cambridge: Cambridge University Press.

Carter, C. O., Evans, K. A., Fraser Roberts, J. A., Buck, A. R. 1971. Genetic clinic follow-up. *Lancet* 1: 281–5.

Cassell, E. J. 1995. Pain and suffering. In: Reich W. (Ed.) *Encyclopedia of Bioethics, 2nd edn*, pp. 1897–1904. New York: Macmillan.

Chadwick, R. 1993. What counts as success in genetic counseling? *J. Med. Ethics* 19: 43–6.

Chadwick, R., Ngwena, C. 1992. The development of a normative standard in counselling for genetic disease: ethics and law. *J. Soc. Welfare Fam. Law* 4: 276–95.

Chadwick, R., ten Have, H., Husted, J. *et al.* 1998. Genetic screening and ethics: European perspectives. *J. Med. Philos.* 23: 255–73.

Chapple, J. C., Dale, R., Evans, B. G. 1987. The new genetic: will it pay its way? *Lancet* i: 1189–92.

Clarke, A. 1990. Genetics, ethics and audit. *Lancet* 335: 1145–7.

  1991. Is non-directive genetic counselling possible? *Lancet* 338: 998–1001.

  1993. Response to: What counts as success in genetic counselling? *J. Med. Ethics* 19: 47–9.

  (Ed.) 1994. *Genetic Counselling. Practice and Principles.* London: Routledge.

  1997*a*. Outcomes and processes in genetic counselling. In: Harper, P. S., Clarke, A. J. (Eds) *Genetics, Society and Clinical Practice*, pp. 165–78. Oxford: BIOS Scientific Publishers.

  1997*b*. The process of genetic counselling: beyond non-directiveness. In: Harper, P. S., Clarke, A. J. *Genetics, Society and Clinical Practice.* Oxford: BIOS Scientific Publishers.

Clarke, A. M., Clarke, D. B., Berg, J. M. (Eds) 1985. *Mental Deficiency: The Changing Outlook.* Cambridge: Methuen and Co.

Conrad, P. 1997. Public eyes and private genes: historical frames, new constructions, and social problems. *Soc. Problems* 44: 139–55.

  2001. Media images, genetics and culture: potential impacts of reporting scientific findings on bioethics. In: Barry Hoffmaster (Ed.) *Bioethics in Social Context*, pp. 90–111. Philadelphia, PA: Temple University Press.

Copel, J. A., Bahado-Singh, R. O. 1999. Prenatal screening for Down's syndrome – a search for the family's values. *New Engl. J. Med.* 341: 521–2.

Coulter, D. L. 1997. Health-related application of quality of life. In: Schalock, R. L., Siperstein, G. N. (Eds) *Quality of Life Volume II. Application to Persons with Disabilities*, pp. 95–104. Washington, DC: American Association on Mental Retardation.

Cowan, R. S. 1994. Women's roles in the history of amniocentesis and chorionic villi sampling. In: Rothenberg, K. H., Thomson, E. J. (Eds) *Women and Prenatal Testing*, pp. 35–48. Columbus, OH: Ohio State University Press.

Cuckle, H. 1998. Rational Down syndrome screening policy. *Am. J. Public Health* 88: 558–9.

Dalgaard, O. Z., Norby, S. 1989. Autosomal dominant polycystic kidney disease in the 1980s. *Clin. Genet.* 36: 320–5.

D'Alton, M. E., DeCherney, A. H. 1993. Prenatal diagnosis. *New Engl. J. Med.* 328: 114–20.

Dodge, J. A. 1998. Gene therapy for cystic fibrosis: what message for the recipient? *Thorax* 53: 157–8.

Downie, R. S., Calman, K. C. 1994. *Healthy Respect. Ethics in Health Care.* Oxford: Oxford University Press.

Durkin, M. S. 1996. Beyond mortality – residential placement and quality of life among children with mental retardation. *Am. J. Public Health* 86: 1359–60.

Ebstein, R. P., Novick, O., Umansky, R. 1996. Dopamine D4 receptor (D4DR) exon III polymorphism associated with the human personality trait of novelty seeking. *Nat. Genet.* 12(Jan): 78–80.

Edgerton, R. B. 1996. A longitudinal ethnographic research perspective on quality of life. In: Schalock, R. L., Siperstein, G. N. (Eds) *Quality of Life Volume I. Conceptualization and Measurement*, pp. 83–90. Washington, DC: American Association on Mental Retardation.

Edwards, S. 1997. The moral status of intellectually disabled individuals. *J. Med. Philos.* 22: 29–42.

Engel, G. 1977. The need for a new medical model: A challenge for biomedicine. *Science* 4286: 129–35.

Engelhardt, H. T. 1986. *The Foundations of Bioethics.* Oxford: Oxford University Press.

Evans, M. 1996. Some ideas of the person. In: Greaves, D., Upton, H. (Eds) *Philosophical Problems in Health Care*, pp. 23–35. Aldershot: Avebury.

Evans, M. I., Hallak, M., Johnson, M. P. 1995. Genetic testing and screening: prenatal diagnosis. In: *The Encyclopedia of Bioethics*, pp. 986–91. New York, NY: Macmillan.

Felce, D., Perry, J. 1996. Assessment of quality of life. In: Schalock, R. L., Siperstein, G. N. (Eds) *Quality of Life Volume I. Conceptualization and Measurement*, pp. 63–72. Washington, DC: American Association on Mental Retardation.

Fricker, J. 1996. PET and obsessive-compulsive disorder. *Lancet* 347: 604.

Friedmann, T. 1990. Opinion: the human genome project – some implications of extensive 'reverse genetic' medicine. *Am. J. Hum. Genet.* 46: 407–14.

Froster, U. G., Jackson, L. 1996. Limb defects and chorionic villus sampling: results from an international registry, 1992–94. *Lancet* 347: 489–94.

Fryers, T. 1984. The epidemiology of severe intellectual impairment. London: Academic Press.
   1992. Epidemiology and taxonomy in mental retardation. *Paediatr. Perinat. Epidemiol.* 6: 181–92.

Gates, E. A. 1994. Prenatal genetic testing: does it benefit pregnant women? In: Rothenberg, K. H., Thomson, E. J. (Eds) *Women and Prenatal Testing*, pp. 183–200. Columbus, OH: Ohio State University Press.

Gath, A. 1990. Down syndrome children and their families. *Am. J. Med. Genet.* 7(Suppl.): 314–16.

Gillam, L. 1999. Prenatal diagnosis and discrimination against the disabled. *J. Med. Ethics* 25: 163–71.

Gillon, R. 1994. *Philosophical Medical Ethics.* Chichester: John Wiley & Sons.

Glass, B. 1971. Science: endless horizons or golden age? *Science* 171: 23–9.

Goodey, C. 1997. Learning difficulties and the guardians of the gene. In: Clarke, A., Parsons, E. (Eds) *Culture, Kinship and Genes*, pp. 206–17. Basingstoke, UK: Macmillan.

Gracia, D. 1993. The intellectual basis of bioethics in Southern European countries. *Bioethics* 7: 97–107.

Gräsbeck, R. 1995. Normaalin käsite lääketieteessä. In: Louhiala, P. Lääketiede ja filosofia, pp. 66–77. Helsinki: Yliopistopaino. (*The concept of normal in medicine.* In Finnish)

Gregg, I. 1994. A memorable patient. Divine intervention? *Br. Med. J.* 309: 928.

Griffin, J. 1986. *Well-being.* Oxford: Clarendon Press.

Grossman, H. J. (Ed.) 1983. *Classification in Mental Retardation (3rd rev.).* Washington, DC: American Association on Mental Deficiency.

Hagberg, G. 1992. Severe and mild mental retardation – the epidemiologists view. *Abstracts of the Congress on Mental Retardation in Childhood, Oslo.*

Hallamaa, J. 1994. *The Prisms of Moral Personhood.* Helsinki: Luther-Agricola-Society.

Hare, R. 1976. Survival of the weakest. In: Gorovitz, S. et al. (Eds) *Moral Problems in Medicine*, pp. 364–9. Englewood Cliffs, NJ: Prentice-Hall.

Harper, P. S., Clarke, A. J. 1997. *Genetics, Society and Clinical Practice*. Oxford: BIOS Scientific Publishers.

Harris, J. 1985. *The Value of Life*. London: Routledge & Kegan Paul.

1998*a. Clones, Genes and Immortality*. Oxford: Oxford University Press.

1998*b*. Should we attempt to eradicate disability? In: Morscher, E. *et al.* (Eds) *Applied Ethics in a Troubled World*, pp. 105–14. Dordrecht: Kluwer.

Hasle, H., Haunstrup Clemmensen, I., Mikkelsen, M. 2000. Risks of leukaemia and solid tumours in individuals with Down's syndrome. *Lancet* 355: 165–9.

Hatton, C. 1998. Whose quality of life is it anyway? Some problems with the emerging quality of life consensus. *Ment. Retard.* 36: 104–15.

Hauerwas, S. 1986. *Suffering Presence. Theological Reflections on Medicine in the Mentally Handicapped and the Church*. Notre Dame: University of Notre Dame Church.

Häyry, H. 1991. *The Limits of Medical Paternalism*. London: Routledge.

Häyry, M. 1990. *Critical Studies in Philosophical Medical Ethics* (Dissertation). Helsinki: University of Helsinki.

Heal, L. W., Sigelman, C. K. 1996. Methodological issues in quality of life measurement. In: Schalock, R. L., Siperstein, G. N. (Eds) *Quality of Life Volume I. Conceptualization and Measurement*, pp. 91–104. Washington, DC: American Association on Mental Retardation.

Hennekens, C. H., Buring, J. E. 1987. *Epidemiology in Medicine*. Boston: Little, Brown and Company.

Herrnstein, R. J. 1994. *The Bell Curve: Intelligence and Class Structure in American Life*. New York: Free Press.

Hietala, M. 1998. *Prospects for Genetic Screening in Finland* (Dissertation). Turku: Annales Universitatis Turkuensis D 322.

Hietala, M., Grön, K., Syvänen, A. -C., Peltonen, L., Aula, P. 1993. Prospects of carrier screening of aspartylglucosaminuria in Finland. *Eur. J. Hum. Genet.* 1: 296–300.

Hill, E. C. 1986. Your morality or mine? An inquiry into the ethics of human reproduction. *Am. J. Obstet. Gynecol.* 154: 1173–80.

Hoedemaekers, R. 1998. *Normative Determinanats of Genetic Screening and Testing* (Ph.D. thesis). Wageningen: Eburon P&L.

Holmes-Siedle, M., Ryynanen, M., Lindenbaum, R. H. 1987. Parental decisions regarding termination of pregnancy following prenatal detection of sex chromosome abnormality. *Prenat. Diagn.* 7: 239–44.

Honderich, T. (Ed.) 1995. *The Oxford Companion to Philosophy*. Oxford: Oxford University Press.

Horgan, J. 1993. Eugenics revisited. *Sci. Am.* June: 92–100.

Hubbard, R. 1986. Eugenics and prenatal testing. *Int. J. Health Serv.* 16: 227–42.

Hughes, C., Hwang, B. 1996. Attempts to conceptualize and measure quality of life. In: Schalock, R. L., Siperstein, G. N. (Eds) *Quality of Life Volume I. Conceptualization and Measurement*, pp. 51–62. Washington, DC: American Association on Mental Retardation.

Hunt, J. 1961. *Intelligence and Experience*. New York: Ronald Press.

Imam, Z. 1994. India bans female feticide. *Br. Med. J.* 309: 428.

Isoniemi, A., Hietala, M., Aula, P., Jalanko, A., Peltonen, L. 1995. Identification of a novel mutation causing aspartylglucosaminuria reveals a mutation hotspot region in the aspartylglucosaminuria gene. *Hum. Mutat.* 5: 318–26.

Itälinna, M., Leinonen, E., Saloviita, T. 1994. Kultakutri karhujen talossa. Kehitysvammaisen lapsen perheen voimavarat ja selviytyminen. Tampere: Kehitysvammaisten tukiliitto. (*The resources of a family with an intellectually disabled child.* In Finnish)

Jallinoja, P. 2001. Genetic screening in maternity care: preventive aims and voluntary choices. *Sociol. Health Illness* 23: 286–307.

Jackson, L. G. 1990. Commentary: Prenatal diagnosis: The magnitude of dysgenic effects is small, the human benefits, great. *Birth* 17: 80.

Jones, S. 1996. *In the Blood. God, Genes and Destiny.* London: Flamingo/Harper Collins.

Julian-Reynier, C., Aurran, Y., Dumaret, A. *et al.* 1995. Attitudes towards Down's syndrome: follow up of a cohort of 280 cases. *J. Med. Gen.* 32: 597–9.

Kääriäinen, R., Piepponen, P., Vaskilampi, T. (Eds) 1985. A multi-disciplinary case-control study of mental retardation and subnormality in low birth cohorts. Kuopion Yliopiston Julkaisuja, Kausanterveystiede, Alkuperäistutkimukset nro 1.

Karjalainen, S., Häyry, H. 1992. Luonnollisesta ja luonnottomasta. *Ajatus* 49: 7–13. (*On the natural and the unnatural.* In Finnish)

Kärki, R. 1998. Lääketiede julkisuudessa. Tampere: Vastapaino. (*Medicine and publicity.* In Finnish)

Kass, L. R. 1985. *Toward a More Natural Science.* New York: The Free Press.

1996. The troubled dream of nature as a moral guide. *Hastings Cent. Rep.* 26 (6): 22–4.

Keith, K. D. 1996. Measuring quality of life across cultures: issues and challenges. In: Schalock, R. L., Siperstein, G. N. (Eds) *Quality of Life Volume I. Conceptualization and Measurement,* pp. 73–82. Washington, DC: American Association on Mental Retardation.

Kent, A. P., Dornan, J. C. 1996. Judgment day in utero. *Lancet* 348 (Suppl II): 16.

Kessler, S., Levine, E. K. 1987. Psychological aspects of genetic counselling. IV. The subjective assessment of probability. *Am. J. Med. Genet.* 28: 361–70.

1989. Psychological aspects of genetic counselling. VI. Critical review of the literature dealing with education and reproduction. *Am. J. Med. Genet.* 34: 340–53.

Khanna, S. K. 1997. Traditions and reproductive technology in an urbanizing north Indian village. *Soc. Sci. Med.* 44: 171–80.

Kingston, H. M. 1994. *ABC of Clinical Genetics.* London: BMJ Publishing Group.

Kishnani, P. S., Sullivan, J. A., Keith Walter, B., Spiridigliozzi, G. A., Doraiswamy, P. M., Rama Krishnan, K. R. 1999. Cholinergic therapy for Down's syndrome. *Lancet* 353: 1064–5.

Kitcher, P. 1997. *The Lives to Come. The Genetic Revolution and Human Possibilities.* Harmondsworth: Penguin.

Kopelman, L. 1984. Respect and the retarded: issues of valuing and labeling. In: Kopelman, L., Moskop, J. C. (Eds) *Ethics and Mental Retardation,* pp. 65–85. Dordrecht: Reidel.

Kopelman, L., Irons, T. G., Kopelman, A. E. 1988. Neonatologists judge the 'Baby Doe' regulations. *New Engl. J. Med.* 318: 677–83.

Kuhse, H., Singer, P. 1985. *Should the Baby Live?* Oxford: Oxford University Press.

Kuppermann, M., Goldberg, J. D., Nease, R. F., Washington, A. E. 1999. Who should be offered prenatal diagnosis? The 35-year old question. *Am. J. Public Health* 89: 160–3.

Kurtz, R. A. 1977. *Social Aspects of Mental Retardation.* Lexington, MA: Lexington Books.

Kusum. 1993. The use of prenatal diagnosis for sex selection; the Indian scene. *Bioethics* 7: 149–65.

Lancet 1982. Editorial. Directive counselling. ii: 368–9.

Lauren, M. 1998. Ihmisen perimä sanomalehden sivuilla. Sosiologian pro gradu-tutkielma, Helsingin yliopisto 1998. (*Human genetic heritage on the pages of a newspaper.* MA thesis, University of Helsinki 1998. In Finnish).

Leonard, C. O., Chase, G. A., Childs, B. 1972. Genetic counseling: a consumer's view. *New Engl. J. Med.* 287: 433–9.

Lewontin, R. 1997. Billions and billions of demons. *New York Rev. Books* Jan 9: 28–32; responses and reply March 6: 50–2.

Lippman, A. 1994. Prenatal genetic testing and screening. Constructing needs and reinforcing inequities. In: Clarke, A. (Ed.) *Genetic Counselling. Practice and Principles,* pp. 142–86. London: Routledge.

   1999. Prenatal diagnosis (letter). *Am. J. Public Health* 89: 1592.

Lippman, A., Wilfond, B. S. 1992. 'Twice-told-stories': Stories about genetic disorders. *Am. J. Hum. Genet.* 51: 936–7.

Littlefield, J. W. 1969. Prenatal diagnosis and therapeutic abortion. *New Engl. J. Med.* 280: 722–3.

Louhiala, P. 1993. Kehitysvammaisuuden perinataaliset tekijät. Jyväskylä: STAKES. Tutkimuksia 30. (*Perinatal factors in mental retardation.* Thesis in Finnish)

Lucassen, A. 1998. Ethical issues in genetic of mental disorders. *Lancet* 352: 1004–5.

Macmillan, D. L., Gresham, F. M., Siperstein, G. N. 1993. Conceptual and psychometric concerns about the 1992 AAMR definition of mental retardation. *Am. J. Ment. Retard.* 98: 325–35.

Marteau, T. M. 1995. Toward informed decisions about prenatal testing: a review. *Prenat. Diagn.* 15: 1215–26.

Marteau, T. M., Drake, H. 1995. Attributions for disability: the influence of genetic screening. *Soc. Sci. Med.* 40: 1127–32.

Marteau, T. M., Kidd, J., Cook, R. *et al.* 1991. Perceived risk not actual risk predicts uptake of amniocentesis. *Br. J. Obstet. Gynecol.* 98: 282–6.

Marteau, T. M., Slack, J., Kidd, J., Shaw, R. 1992. Presenting a routine screening test in antenatal care: practice observed. *Public Health* 106: 131–41.

Marteau, T. M., Drake, H., Bobrow, M. 1994*a*. Counselling following diagnosis of fetal abnormality; the differing approaches of obstetricians, clinical geneticists and genetic nurses. *J. Med. Genet.* 31: 864–7.

Marteau, T. M., Drake, H., Reid, M. 1994*b*. Counselling following diagnosis of fetal abnormality: a comparison between German, Portuguese and UK geneticists. *Eur. J. Hum. Genet.* 2: 96–102.

Matikka, L. 2000. Comparability of quality-of-life-studies of the general population and people with intellectual disabilities. *Scand. J. Disabil. Res.* 2: 83–102.

Matikka, L., Vesala, H. T. 1997. Acquiescence in quality-of-life interviews with adults who have mental retardation. *Ment. Retard.* 35: 75–82.

Mayor, S. 1999. Parents of people with Down's syndrome report suboptimal case. *Br. Med. J.* 318: 687.

McCullough, L. B. 1984. The world gained and the world lost: labeling the mentally retarded. In: Kopelman, L., Moskop, J. C. (Eds) *Ethics and Mental Retardation*, pp. 99–118. Dordrecht: Reidel.

McGuffin, P., Thapar, A. 1997. Genetic basis of bad behaviour in adolescents. *Lancet* 350: 411–12.

McLaughlin, J. F., Bjornson, K. F. 1998. Quality of life and developmental disabilities. *Dev. Med. Child Neurol.* 40: 435.

Michie, S., Bron, F., Bobrow, M., Marteau, T. M. 1997*a*. Nondirectivenes in genetic counselling: an empirical study. *Am. J. Hum. Genet.* 60: 40–7.

Michie, S., Marteau, T. M., Bobrow, M. 1997*b*. Genetic counselling: the psychological impact of meeting patients' expectations. *J. Med. Genet.* 34: 237–41.

Modell, B., Kuliev, A. M. 1991. Services for thalassemia as a model for cost–benefit analysis of genetic services. *J. Inherit. Metabol. Dis.* 14: 640–51.

Molenaar, J. C. 1992. A Report from the Netherlands. The legal investigation of a decision not to operate on an infant with Down's syndrome and duodenal atresia. *Bioethics* 6: 35–40.

Munthe, C. 1996. *The Moral Roots of Prenatal Diagnosis. Studies in Research Ethics No 7.* Göteborg: The Royal Society of Arts and Sciences in Gotherburg, Centre for Research Ethics.

Murphy, T. F. 1985. The moral significance of spontaneous abortion. *J. Med. Ethics* 11: 79–83.

Murray, J., Cuckle, H., Taylor, G., Hewison, J. 1997. Screening for fragile X syndrome: information needs for health planners. *J. Med. Screening* 4: 60–94.

Musschenga, A. W. 1997. The relation between concepts of quality-of-life, health and happiness. *J. Med. Philos.* 22: 11–28.

Nature 1991. Editorial: Ethics and the human genome. 351: 591.

Nat. Genet. 1997. Editorial: Brave new now. 15: 1–2.

Nelkin, D., Lindee, M. S. 1995. *The DNA Mystique. The Gene as a Cultural Icon.* New York: W. H. Freeman and Company.

Nelkin, D., Tancredi, L. 1995. Health screening and testing in the public-health context. In: Reich, W. (Ed.) *Encyclopedia of Bioethics*, pp. 1129–32. New York: Macmillan.

Nesse, R. M., Williams, G. C. 1994. *Why We Get Sick. The New Science of Darwinian Medicine.* New York: Times Books, Random House.

Nicholson, A., Alberman, E. 1992. Cerebral palsy – an increasing contributor to severe mental retardation? *Arch. Dis. Child.* 67: 1050–5.

Nielsen, B. B., Liljestrand, J., Hedegaard, M., Thilsted, S. H., Joseph, A. 1997. Reproductive pattern, perinatal mortality, and sex preference in rural Tamil Nadu, south India: community based, cross sectional study. *Br. Med. J.* 314: 1521–4.

Noddings, N. 1984. *Caring. A Feminine Approach to Ethics and Moral Education.* Berkeley: University of California Press.

Nordenfelt, L. 1987. *On the Nature of Health. An Action – Theoretic Approach.* Dordrecht: Reidel.

Palo, J. 1995. Ei ihan tavalliset ihmiset. Helsingin Sanomat Kuukausiliite 25: 46–50. (*Not just ordinary people.* In Finnish)

Palomaki, G. E. 1994. Population based prenatal screening for the fragile X syndrome. *J. Med. Screen.* 1: 65–72.

Palomaki, G. E., Haddow, J. E. 1996. Is it time for population-based prenatal screening for fragile-X? *Lancet* 341: 373–4.

Parens, E. 1996. Taking behavioral genetics seriously. *Hastings Cent. Rep.* 26(4): 13–22.

Parfit, D. 1976. Rights, interests and possible people. In: Gorovitz, S. *et al.* (Eds) *Moral Problems in Medicine*, pp. 369–75. Englewood Cliffs, NJ: Prentice-Hall.

Parsons, E. 1997. Culture and genetics: is genetics in society or society in genetics? In: Clarke, A., Parsons, E. (Eds) *Culture, Kinship and Genes*. Basingstoke, UK: Macmillan.

Parsons, E., Bradley, D. 1994. Ethical issues in newborn screening for Duchenne muscular dystrophy. In: Clarke, A. (Ed.) *Genetic Counselling. Practice and Principles*, pp. 95–112. London: Routledge.

Pauker, S. P., Pauker, S. G. 1994. Prenatal diagnosis – why is 35 a magical number? *New Engl. J. Med.* 330: 1151–2.

Payer, L. 1990. *Medicine and Culture*. London: Victor Gollancz.

Peippo, M. 1995. FraX-oireyhtymän perinnöllisyys. In: Arvio, M., Laine, P. (Eds) FraX-oireyhtymä pojalla ja miehellä. Pääjärven kuntayhtymän tutkimusraportti, pp. 6–13. (*Heritability of FraX syndrome*. In Finnish)

Powledge, T., Fletcher, J. 1979. Guidelines for the ethical, social and legal issues in prenatal diagnosis. *New Engl. J. Med.* 300: 168–72.

Press, N. A., Browner, C. H. 1994. Collective silences, collective fictions: how prenatal diagnostic testing became part of routine prenatal care. In: Rothenberg, K. H., Thomsen, E. J. (Eds) *Women and Prenatal Testing*, pp. 201–18. Columbus: Ohio State University Press.

1997. Why women say yes to prenatal diagnosis. *Soc. Sci. Med.* 45: 979–89.

Pueschel, S. M. 1990. Clinical aspects of Down syndrome from infancy to adulthood. *Am. J. Med. Genet.* Suppl. 7: 52–6.

Puskala, R. M. 1995. In: Reinikka–Tevalin, R. (Ed.) *Sikiödiagnostiikka – näkökulmia*, pp. 40–3. Tampere: Kehitysvammaisten tulikiiton IKI – instituntti. (*Fetal diagnosis – points of view*. In Finnish)

Qureshi, N. 1997. The relevance of cultural understanding to clinical genetic practice. In: Clarke, A., Parsons, E. (Eds) *Culture, Kinship and Genes*, pp. 111–19. Basingstoke, UK: Macmillan.

Rantakallio, P., von Wendt, L. 1986. Mental retardation and subnormality in a birth cohort of 12000 children in Northern Finland. *Am. J. Ment. Defic.* 90: 380–7.

Rapp, R. 1994. Women's responses to prenatal diagnosis: a sociocultural perspective on diversity. In: Rothenberg, K. H., Thomson, E. J. (Eds) *Women and Prenatal Testing*, pp. 219–33. Columbus, OH: Ohio State University Press.

Reid, M. 1991. The diffusion of four prenatal screening tests across Europe. London: King's Fund Centre for Health Services Development.

Richardson, M. K., Reiss, M. J. 1999. What does the human embryo look like, and does it matter? *Lancet* 354: 244–6.

Richardson, S. A., Koller, H. 1985. Epidemiology. In: Clarke, A. M., Clarke, D. B., Berg, J. M. (Eds) *Mental Deficiency: The Changing Outlook*, pp. 356–400. Cambridge: Methuen and Co.

Rose, G. 1992. *The Strategy of Preventive Medicine*. Oxford: Oxford University Press.

Rose, S. 1995. The rise of neurogenetic determinism. *Nature* 373: 380–2.

Rose-Ackerman, S. 1982. Mental retardation and society: The ethics and politics of normalization. *Ethics* 93: 81–101.

Rosen, M., Clark, G. R., Kivitz, M. S. (Eds) 1976. *The History of Mental Retardation. Collected Papers.* Baltimore: University Park Press.

Rothman, B. K. 1994. The tentative pregnancy: then and now. In: Rothenberg, K. H., Thomson, E. J. (Eds) *Women and Prenatal Testing*, pp. 260–70. Columbus, OH: Ohio State University Press.

Rowley, P. T., Loader, S., Sutera, C. J., Walden, M. 1989. Do pregnant women benefit form hemoglobinopathy carrier detection? *Ann. N. Y. Acad. Sci.* 565: 152–60.

Santalahti, P., Hemminki, E. 1998. Use of prenatal screening tests in Finland. *Eur. J. Public Health* 8: 8–14.

Santalahti, P., Latikka, A. M., Ryynänen, M., Hemminki, E. 1996. Women's experiences of prenatal serum screening. *Birth* 23: 101–7.

Santalahti, P., Hemminki, E., Latikka, A. M., Ryynänen, M. 1998. Women's decision-making in prenatal screening. *Soc. Sci. Med.* 46: 1067–76.

Schalock, R. L. 1996. Reconsidering the conceptualization and measurement of quality of life. In: Schalock, R. L., Siperstein, G. N. (Eds) *Quality of Life Volume I. Conceptualization and Measurement*, pp. vii–xi. Washington, DC: American Association on Mental Retardation.

Siperstein, G. N. (Eds) 1996. *Quality of Life Volume I. Conceptualization and Measurement.* Washington, DC: American Association on Mental Retardation.

(Eds) 1997. *Quality of Life Volume II. Application to Persons with Disabilities.* Washington, DC: American Association on Mental Retardation.

Schwartz, K. 1976. Nature's corrective principle in social evolution. Original 1908, reprinted in Rosen, M., Clark, G. R., Kivitz, M. S. (Eds) 1976. *The History of Mental Retardation. Collected Papers*, vol. 2, pp. 147–63. Baltimore: University Park Press.

Schwartz, R. 1996. Genetic knowledge: Some legal and ethical questions. In: Thomasma, D. C., Kushner, T. (Eds) *Birth to Death. Science and Bioethics*, pp. 21–34. Cambridge: Cambridge University Press.

Sen, A. 1993. Capability and well-being. In: Nussbaum, M. C., Sen, A. (Eds) *The Quality of Life*, pp. 30–53. Oxford: Clarendon Press.

Serra-Prat, M., Gallo, P., Jovell, A. J., Aymerich, M., Estrada, M. D. 1998. Trade-offs in prenatal detection of Down syndrome. *Am. J. Public Health* 88: 551–7.

Sheldon, T. 1999. Dutch doctors call for all pregnant women to be screened for Down's. *Br. Med. J.* 319: 872.

Shepperdson, B. 1983. Abortion and euthanasia of Down's syndrome children – the parents' view. *J. Med. Ethics* 9: 152–7.

Simola, K. 1995. Sikiötutkimukset – mitä, kenelle ja miksi? In: Reinikka-Tevalin, R. Sikiödiagnostiikka – näkökulmia, pp. 7–13. Tampere: Kehitysvammaisten tulikiiton IKI-instituutti. (*Fetal investigations – what, to whom and why?* In Finnish)

Simpson, J. L. 1991. Screening for fetal and genetic abnormalities. *Baillière's Clin. Obstet. Gynaecol.* 5: 675–96.

Singer, P. 1993. *Practical Ethics.* Cambridge: Cambridge University Press.

Sjögren, B., Uddenberg, N. 1988. Decision making during the prenatal diagnostic procedure. A questionnaire and interview study of 211 women participating in prenatal diagnosis. *Prenat. Diagn.* 8: 263–73.

Skeels, H. M., Dye, H. B. 1976. A study of the effects of differential stimulation on mentally retarded children. Original 1939, reprinted in Rosen, M., Clark, G. R., Kivitz, M. S. (Eds) *The History of Mental Retardation. Collected Papers*, vol. 2, pp. 241–66. Baltimore: University Park Press.

Smith, D. K., Shaw, R. W., Marteau, T. M. 1994. Informed consent to undergo screening for Down's syndrome: the gap between policy and practice. *Br. Med. J.* 309: 776.

Somer, M., Mustonen, H., Norio, R. 1988. Evaluation of genetic counseling: Recall of information, post-counseling reproduction, and attitude of the counsellees. *Clin. Genet.* 34: 352–65.

Spallone, P. 1997. 'Once you have a hammer, everything looks like a nail'. In: Clarke, A., Parsons, E. (Eds) *Culture, Kinship and Genes*, pp. 197–205. Basingstoke: Macmillan.

Sternberg, R. J. 1990. *Metaphors of Mind – Conceptions of the Nature of Intelligence*. Cambridge: Cambridge University Press.

Strauss, D., Eyman, R. K., Grossman, H. J. 1996. Predictors of mortality in children with severe mental retardation: the effect of placement. *Am. J. Public Health* 86: 1422–9.

Sutton, A. 1990. *Prenatal Diagnosis: Confronting the Ethical Issues*. London: The Linacre Centre.

Taylor, S. J., Bogdan, R. 1996. Quality of life and the individual's perspective. In: Schalock, R. L., Siperstein, G. N. (Eds) *Quality of Life Volume I. Conceptualization and Measurement*, pp. 11–22. Washington, DC: American Association on Mental Retardation.

The Danish Council of Ethics. 1993. *Ethics and Mapping of the Human Genome*. Copenhagen: Danish Council of Ethics.

Tooley, M. 1972. Abortion and infanticide. *Philos. Public Affairs* 2: 37–65.

Vácha, J. 1982. The problem of so-called normality in anthropological sciences. *Modern Man, Anthropos (Brno)* 22: 73–85.

Vanhatalo, S. 1999. Sikiön kipu – totta vai yliempaattista kuvittelua? Duodecim 115: 1458–63. (*Foetal pain – true or imagination?* In Finnish)

Vehmas, S. 1999*a*. Discriminative assumptions of utilitarian bioethics regarding individuals with intellectual disabilities. *Disabil. Soc.* 14: 37–52.

    1999*b*. Newborn infants and the moral significance of intellectual disabilities. *J. Assoc. Persons Sev. Handicaps* 24: 111–21.

Virkkula, S. 1998. Karsi vammaisia, karsit kuluja. *Aamulehti* 26. 4. 1998: 17–18 (*Less disabled, less costs*. In Finnish)

Wald, N. J., Kennard, A., Hackshaw, A., McGuire, A. 1997. Antenatal screening for Down's syndrome. *J. Med. Screen.* 4: 181–246.

Warren, M. A. 1997. *Moral Status. Obligations to Persons and Other Living Things*. Oxford: Clarendon Press.

Watson, E., Mayall, E., Chapple, J. *et al.* 1991. Carrier screening for cystic fibrosis. *Br. Med. J.* 303: 405–7.

Watson, J. 1997–1998. Good gene, bad gene. What is the right way to fight the tragedy of genetic disease? *Time*, Special issue, Winter: 86.

Welie, J. V. M. 1998. *In the Face of Suffering. The Philosophical-Anthropological Foundations of Clinical Ethics*. Omaha: Creighton University Press.

Wertz, D. 1997. Reconsidering 'nondirectiveness' in genetic counseling. *Gene Letter* 1, Issue 4 (http://www.geneletter.org/0197/counseling.htm)

Wertz, D., Fletcher, J. C. 1988. Attitude of genetic counselors: a multinational survey. *Am. J. Hum. Genet.* 42: 592–600.

White, M. T. 1998. Decision-making through dialogue: reconfiguring autonomy in genetic counseling. *Theoret. Med. Bioethics* 19: 5–19.

  1999. Making responsible decisions. An interpretive ethic for genetic decision making. *Hastings Cent. Rep.* 29: 14–21.

Whitten, C. F. 1973. Sickle-cell programming – an imperiled promise. *New Engl. J. Med.* 288: 318–19.

Wickelgren, I. 1999. Nurture helps mold able minds. *Science* 283: 1832–4.

Wilska, M. 2001. Aina syntyy lapsia, joiden vammaisuus tulee yllätyksenä. Helsingin Sanomat. (*There will always be children whose disability will be a surprise.* In Finnish)

Wolraich, M. L., Siperstein, G. N., Reed, D. 1991. Doctors' decisions and prognostications for infants with Down syndrome. *Dev. Med. Child Neurol.* 33: 336–42.

World Health Organization 1980. *International Classification of Impairments, Disabilities and Handicaps.* Geneva: WHO.

Wulff, H., Andur Pedersen, S., Rosenberg, R. 1986. *Philosophy of Medicine – An Introduction.* Oxford: Blackwell.

Zigler, E., Balla, D., Hodapp, R. 1984. On the definition and classification of mental retardation. *Am. J. Ment. Defic.* 89: 215–30.

Index

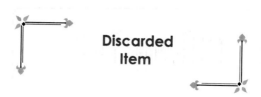

Discarded Item